COLORFUL KETO

It's About More Than Weight Loss

COLORFUL KETO

It's About More Than Weight Loss

YOUR SUSTAINABLE KETOGENIC DIET AND LIFESTYLE GUIDE

NICOLE QUEZADA, CNC

PUBLISHING & COPYRIGHT

COLORFUL KETO
IT'S ABOUT MORE THAN WEIGHT LOSS

COPYRIGHT © 2024 GROWING FORWARD PRODUCTIONS, LLC

ALL RIGHT RESERVED
NO PORTION OF THIS BOOK MAY BE REPRODUCED, STORED IN A RETRIEVAL SYSTEM, OR TRANSMITTED IN ANY FORM OR BY ANY MEANS - ELECTRONIC, MECHANICAL, PHOTOCOPIED, RECORDING, SCANNING, OR OTHER - EXCEPT FOR BRIEF QUOTATIONS IN REVIEWS OR ARTICLES WITHOUT PRIOR WRITTEN PERMISSION OF THE PUBLISHER.

PUBLISHED IN ATLANTA, GA, BY BE A BETTER ME

DISCLAIMER
I AM NOT A DOCTOR, NURSE, MEDICAL PROFESSIONAL, OR REGISTERED DIETITIAN, NOR DO I CLAIM TO BE. THE INFORMATION IS FOR EDUCATIONAL PURPOSES ONLY. RECOMMENDATIONS OF BEHAVIORS OR PRODUCTS ARE NOT INTENDED TO DIAGNOSE OR CURE DISEASE. THIS BOOK IS BASED ON SCIENTIFIC STUDIES AND MY PERSONAL EXPERIENCE AS A NUTRITION AND FITNESS PROFESSIONAL. I DO NOT GUARANTEE THAT YOU WILL ATTAIN A SPECIFIC RESULT. PLEASE COORDINATE WITH YOUR HEALTHCARE PROVIDER BEFORE STARTING ANY NEW DIET OR EXERCISE PROGRAM. I EXPLICITLY DISCLAIM RESPONSIBILITY TO ANY PERSON OR ENTITY FOR ANY LIABILITY, LOSS, OR DAMAGE CAUSED OR ALLEGED TO BE CAUSED DIRECTLY OR INDIRECTLY DUE TO THE USE, APPLICATION, OR INTERPRETATION OF ANY MATERIAL PROVIDED IN THIS BOOK.

ISBN: 979-8-218-42472-5 - PAPERBACK
ISBN: 979-8-218-51857-8 - EBOOK

COVER DESIGN & INTERIOR DESIGN BY:
NICOLE QUEZADA

Dedication

To my mom, who showed me that you are never too old to change your health.

To my clients, thank you for continually showing up for yourself and me.

To all those who seek to change their health and not repeat the same patterns of those who came before you.

CONTENTS

HEALTH STRUGGLES
1

INTRODUCTION
1

CHAPTER 1: DISPELLING THE MYTH
3

CHAPTER 2: UNVEILING THE HEALTH BENEFITS
9

CHAPTER 3: OUR METABOLIC HEALTH CRISIS
17

CHAPTER 4: BASIC KETO PRINCIPLES
23

CHAPTER 5: GETTING STARTED
29

CHAPTER 6: NAVIGATING CHALLENGES
49

CHAPTER 7: EMBRACING THE KETOGENIC LIFESTYLE
55

CONCLUSION
63

RESOURCES
67

HEALTH STRUGGLES NO, EVERYTHING IS NOT "NORMAL"

When I first heard about the ketogenic diet in 2016, I assumed it was another fad diet that would disappear after a few years. Based on the USDA's nutritional guidelines (MyPlate), I ate what I thought was healthy. I wasn't a big sweet eater because diabetes runs on both sides of my family. I did, however, love my pasta, grains, vegetables, and fruits. I had no interest in pulling those things out of my diet, so I ignored everything else I heard about the diet for quite a few years.

Fast forward to 2019, in my late 30s. I realized I had been having clarity and focus issues for a few years, and I felt it was progressively getting worse. I wasn't sleeping well, and I lacked energy more and more each day. I found myself feeling run down and even depressed at times. I knew that all these things weren't "normal" for me. I had gained a few extra pounds over the years that wouldn't seem to come off either, which was frustrating. I was getting my yearly physicals regularly, and the doctor said all my blood work was good and that she didn't see any issues. I discussed all of the problems that I was having, and she did perform one extra test on my thyroid, but just like everything else, it came back as being within the normal ranges.

None of this made sense to me. How could I have all these issues in my life and be told by my doctor that everything was normal? I asked her what she thought might be causing all the issues that I was experiencing. I was told it might be stress-related or some early onset pre-menopause because I didn't have kids. Now, seriously, I was like, *"What the heck? I'm only 39 years old; surely that can't be right?"*

I knew that there had to be something I could do with my nutrition and exercise to help this situation. I dove head first into researching these things online. You don't realize how much information is out there about food, diet, and exercise until you start looking for it. How is someone supposed to know what's true and what's not? It can be so overwhelming. I decided to focus on one thing at a time. I started with exercise because I have always heard *"eat less and move more."* After a few weeks, not much changed. I was still unfocused, having sleep and clarity issues, and hadn't lost any weight. I didn't understand that exercise doesn't work on its own. It must be paired with proper nutritional changes to induce changes.

I was still eating what I thought was healthy—mainly the Standard American Diet (S.A.D. for short) with fewer carbs than they suggested. Again, I dove into the internet, researching diet information and different eating methods that might help alleviate my symptoms. The ketogenic diet kept coming up in those searches as a way to reduce or even get rid of the symptoms that I was experiencing. I kept saying, *"No, that goes against everything I know about nutrition and everything I have ever been taught about nutrition. How could this be good for me?"*

One evening, I was at home listening to a podcast and heard something I will never forget. I will paraphrase here, but the person on the podcast said, *"If you only read and research about things that validate your current opinion, how do you know it's actually your opinion?"* This blew my mind, and I related that to my nutrition. I started questioning everything I knew (or thought I knew) and was taught about nutrition up to that point. I became open to the ketogenic diet and the benefits that I could gain from it.

I asked myself, *"If I tried this for 30 days, would it kill me?"* Based on my research up to that point, "*NO*," it wouldn't, so what could it hurt to give it a try? In January 2020, I did my first strict keto phase for 28 days, which changed my mind and life.

I not only started losing weight in the first week, but after about five days, I started sleeping well again. I didn't get hangry if I didn't have food within two to three hours of my last meal. I felt fuller from much smaller amounts of food. I gained focus and clarity that I had never experienced before in my entire life. I had lots of energy throughout the day and stopped experiencing the afternoon slump I was so accustomed to. I had suffered from migraines since my teenage years, some years having as many as twelve per year to only having two or three per year. I wanted to be more active and try things I had never even thought about before, from different and new foods to new types of exercises. My overall well-being and drive to learn new things went through the roof. I felt like I was a more intelligent person. I'm unsure if that is real, but I felt so good that it was invigorating. When I say that my mind and life changed, it did, and all of these beautiful benefits continue today even after four years of living this ketogenic lifestyle.

I previously mentioned that diabetes runs on both sides of my family, specifically type 2 diabetes. My father, mother, brother, and one of my grandmothers suffered from it. My mother, by the grace of god, decided to change her story.

In late 2020, my mother needed to have knee replacement surgery. Before this, I worked with her on lifestyle and nutrition changes. She stopped eating out two to three times a day and started eating at home; she reduced her stress levels by retiring from work, and she started taking some vitamins and other supplements that allowed her to stop taking high blood pressure and high cholesterol medications (statin medications). However, she was still on medication for diabetes because her A1C level averaged 6.7 while on medications. When she went in to see her surgeon. He told her that for him to perform the surgery, she had to lose at least 20 lbs. She came to me that day and said, *"Ok, I'm ready to try this keto thing. I have to lose this weight so I can get this surgery."* Of course, I said, *"Let's do it, mom!"*

We started her on the ketogenic diet the next day. Four weeks later, she had lost 20 pounds, an average weight loss in the first month if someone is obese and stays strict with their keto diet. Her doctor scheduled the surgery. She continued the diet for the next few months, and a few months after her surgery, she went to her primary care doctor. Her doctor told her that her A1C numbers were showing in the normal range (between 5.4 and 6.4) and that they wanted to start reducing her diabetes medication (metformin). The doctor asked her what she had been doing, and she told her that she had been doing the keto diet. While the doctor wasn't thrilled, her numbers looked good, so she told her to stick with it. About eight weeks later, she was taking a quarter of the amount of medication that she was on before she started keto. On her next visit, she was told that she could stop taking the drug but to keep monitoring her blood glucose levels just to be safe. After being diabetic for 13 years, she was no longer a diabetic at the age of 73!

My mom is now 76, and while she doesn't live a ketogenic lifestyle now, she does live a low-carb lifestyle. For her, the diet was a temporary solution that got her back on track to optimal metabolic health. She is happy and healthy and remains free of diabetes to this day!

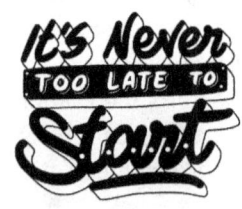

INTRODUCTION

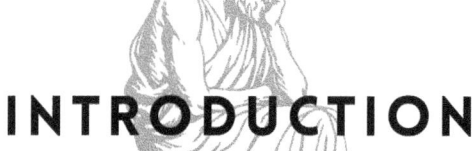

"Let food be thy medicine and medicine be thy food."
- Hippocrates

I'm writing this book as a ketogenic diet and lifestyle practitioner and health and fitness professional. The ketogenic diet has changed my life, my mother's life, and several millions of people worldwide after hundreds of years of use. With all the spectacular ways that the ketogenic diet has transformed my life, I feel it would be a disservice if I didn't share my experience and knowledge with others so that they can benefit from this way of life, too.

Since I have adopted the ketogenic lifestyle, it has changed the way I feel, look, and think. I have continued to research, read, and consume as much as I can about its history, use in the medical field, and use in everyday life to help people improve their health, wellness, and longevity. Keto isn't just a diet; it is a lifestyle. It's a lifestyle that can change your life, too!

A specific keto diet variation that will work for me may not work for you. In all honesty, some people's systems may not work with certain ketogenic variations. Each keto variation should be slightly different because each person's carbohydrate intolerance is different. I'm sure you're saying, *"Great, now I have to figure out which variation might work for me?"* The good news is that is one of the other reasons why I am writing this book.

I aim to provide educational information to help you navigate this process because I remember how hard it was when I first started to find a simple, short (less than 90 pages), all-in-one guide about the ketogenic diet and lifestyle. I will dispel the myth that the ketogenic diet is a fad diet or that it is unsustainable. I will explain all the incredible health benefits outside of weight loss. I'll provide research and information about our current worldwide metabolic health crises. I'll answer the major questions on what you need to do to start the ketogenic way of life. I'll walk you through common challenges, and lastly, I'll provide you with ways to make it sustainable.

I want this to be a ketogenic lifestyle guide and a catalyst to help you improve your life and longevity. Suppose you are interested in finding ways to decrease or even possibly eliminate your risks of having cardiovascular disease or a stroke, mental illness, epilepsy, autoimmune diseases, hypertension, type 2 diabetes, fatty liver disease, some cancers, Amyotrophic lateral sclerosis (ALS), Parkinson's disease, Alzheimer's disease, or polycystic ovary syndrome (PCOS), to name a few studied and researched health issues that the ketogenic diet has been found to help. In that case, you'll want to keep reading.

QUICK NOTE: This is an omnivore-based ketogenic lifestyle book. I will discuss animal—and plant-based foods. A few vegetarians can adopt many of the ideas discussed in this book. Unfortunately, this book doesn't contain dietary information for my vegan friends.

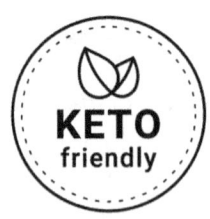

CHAPTER 1: DISPELLING THE MYTH

Many people classify the ketogenic diet as a "fad" diet. So, let's define the word fad before jumping into this short history lesson. Oxford Languages defines a fad as an intense and widely shared enthusiasm for something, especially short-lived and without a basis. Our brief history lesson will dispel the myth that the ketogenic diet is short-lived or without a basis.

> **"Those who do not learn the history are doomed to repeat it." - George Santayana**

The ketogenic diet didn't just pop up in the 1920s for medical use like I thought at one time. Technically, the ketogenic diet has been around since humans have walked the Earth. There was a time when we consumed whole animals and fish (meat, fat, organs, bone & bone marrow), bugs, eggs, minimal amounts of fruits (based on seasonal availability), nuts, seeds, bark, and flowers. This diet gave rise to the term "hunter-gatherer." Carbohydrates only became a common part of the human diet around 10,000 years ago, and processed sugar and flour weren't introduced until 300 years ago.

The first documented use of the ketogenic diet for medical purposes that I found was in the late 1790s by a doctor named

John Rollo. Dr. Rollo used the diet to treat two patients who had diabetes. It is unclear if it was type 1 or type 2 diabetes; nonetheless, it was implemented as a dietary approach to treat the disease since medications were unavailable.

There are accounts of people using the ketogenic diet in the 1800s and early 1900s as well. I'd like to tell you about the first of two early documented practitioners, William Banting. In the 1860s, Mr. Banting started on a weight loss journey, eventually losing over 50 pounds and 13 inches when he was 66. He wrote a public announcement pamphlet back in 1863 called "*Letter on Corpulence, Addressed to the Public*," where he spoke about his weight loss journey implementing the keto diet. He described what he was eating and how it was making him feel. It wasn't the exact keto diet we know today, but it is similar and a variation of the diet.

In the 1920s, it started to get interesting. The second keto practitioner is Vilhjalmur Stefansson. He was a student and later a professor at Harvard. He is best known for his work in anthropology, specifically with the Inuit of the Antarctic. He attended several expeditions to study the diets and lifestyles of Arctic people in the early 1900s. Later in the 1920s, after a few expeditions and experimenting with high-fat food sources, he and another explorer vowed to prove all the doctors wrong about how humans couldn't live optimally without consuming plants. This was the first (unofficial) clinical trial of the ketogenic diet. They vowed to eat only meat and drink water for a year. They were medically observed and given steak, roast beef, brains, tongue, and liver to eat. Stefansson became ill once that year when the researchers instructed him to eat lean meats instead of fatty meats. The sickness disappeared when fat was incorporated back into his diet. The physicians and Stefansson learned that the fat content of the meat was more important than the meat itself. They found the ideal ratio to be three parts fat and one part meat. They continued with the experiment for the entire year. Both men survived, felt great, and were healthy at the end of the experiment. This 3:1 ratio is a ratio of one of the versions of the ketogenic diet we know today.

The ketogenic diet was still being used to manage diabetes in the 1920s, and it was just being introduced as a treatment for epileptic seizures in children by Dr. Russel Wilder of the Mayo Clinic. Dr. Wilder coined the term "ketogenic diet" in 1921. At that time, the ketogenic diet was the most prominent treatment used for seizures in childhood epilepsy and the management of type 1 diabetes.

In 1922, pharmaceutical companies grew and started developing medications to help manage diabetes and epileptic seizures. The use of the ketogenic diet began to dwindle in favor of the medicines because they were promoted as an "easier" way to control these illnesses. After the medications became mainstream, the ketogenic diet was moved to the bottom of the list of treatment options, and only a select few dietitians were trained in its use after this time.

In the early 1930s, Dr. Otto Warburg, a physiologist and medical doctor, won the Nobel Prize for discovering that cancer cells need glucose from carbohydrates to grow and that without it, they will starve to death. Between the prevalence of diabetes and the discovery that cancer cells need glucose to grow, endocrinologists' textbooks started instructing that carbohydrates should be limited and that sugars should be removed from the diet to help reduce the prevalence of these diseases. This vocabulary was later removed without any explanation.

During the period from the 1940s to the mid-1950s, the ketogenic diet seemed to get little attention, but many doctors and everyday people were still using it. In the 1940s, Dr. Blake Donaldson used the diet with thousands of patients and got excellent health and weight loss results. Dr. Alred Pennington heard Dr. Donaldson speak at a conference in the 1950s and started implementing it with Dupont workers with greater success than he had with any other diet intervention. They published articles and books on their work and outcomes from the 1940s through the 1950s. Vince Gironda, a world-famous bodybuilder and trainer, promoted a ketogenic diet for his clients. He believed that sugar and too many carbs were terrible for the body. He recommended that his trainees eat eggs and meat for breakfast, lunch, and dinner and one small carb-rich meal every third to fifth day.

In the mid-1960s, a cardiologist named Dr. Robert Atkins gained inspiration from Dr. Pennington's work. Dr. Atkins tried the diet himself and tried it with 65 executives, who all saw significant weight loss and increased health markers. In 1972, Dr. Atkins introduced the Atkins Diet. He published his first book on the diet titled *Dr. Atkins' Diet Revolution.* This same year, a British professor of nutrition named John Yudkin published a book called *Pure, White, and Deadly*, which was about the dangers of sugar in our diet and how the consumption of it was the leading cause of obesity and heart disease. This was the time when the ketogenic diet started to take hold...right before some overly biased scientific research came out.

Big pharma, big agriculture, and big box brands tried to stamp out the ketogenic diet by paying for studies to conclude that red meats, butter, and eggs, among other healthy fats, were terrible for you and that high cholesterol caused heart disease. To this day, no concrete scientific proof or random control trials prove this. See the resource section for more on this.

Between 1973 and 1991, there were very few publications concerning the ketogenic diet in the medical field or mainstream media due to its stamp out. In 1992, Dr. Atkins released an updated book titled *Dr. Atkins' New Diet Revolution.*

In 1993, a young boy by the name of Charlie had intractable generalized seizures. This means that medications could not control his epileptic seizures. His family was desperate to find something to help him. They stumbled upon some research about the ketogenic diet in a local library. With the partnership and guidance from Charlie's doctor, they started him on the diet. Within a matter of days, they saw improvement. After a month, he was wholly seizure-free and drug-free. Charlie remained on the ketogenic diet for five years. After this time, he was taken off the diet. He can eat whatever he wants and remains drug-free and seizure-free to this day. His parents started a non-profit organization called the Charlie Foundation For Ketogenic Therapies in 1994.

1995 to 2002 was quiet, though doctors and scientists were still researching the diet. Many everyday people were still practicing forms of the diet through the Adkins diet. Dr. Atkins introduced "net carbs" (see Chapter 7 for the definition) in 2002 and updated his book *Dr. Atkins' Diet Revolution* to reflect this. This book has sold over 15 million copies and is considered one of the best-selling diet books ever. This same year, a New York Times article by journalist Gary Taubes was published, and it was called *"What If It's All Been A Big Fat Lie?"* Dr. Atkins' book and this article by Gary Taubes launched the ketogenic and low-carb lifestyle back into the mainstream.

Fast forward 13 years, between 2015 and 2018, there was a 180% increase in online searches about the ketogenic diet based on Google Trends data. In 2021, it had the third place popularity spot for the most searched diet of the year. It's now 2024, and we have over 234 years of documentation on the ketogenic diet. It is still around and still changing people's lives every day.

Next, we will discuss some of the health benefits of this incredible way of living, and I will introduce you to some of the top doctors and researchers in the field.

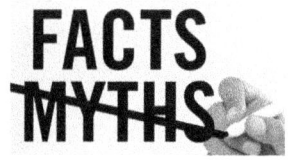

CHAPTER 2: UNVEILING THE HEALTH BENEFITS

People tend to only think about weight loss when they hear about the ketogenic diet or keto for short. For many people, it is one tool for weight loss. For others, it can be a life-changing dietary change for their health, and in many cases, it is both. Some people will lose weight fast, some slow. It all depends on each person's metabolic health and carbohydrate intolerance.

Some people may not lose much scale weight, yet they lose inches, and their health markers improve significantly. The main thing to understand is that this is not a quick-fix diet. In most cases, we did not gain extra weight or get metabolically sick quickly; making these changes will take some time. The amount of time it takes will vary for each person. It is a lifestyle change that will take consistency and dedication to achieve the results you desire.

On the next page, I am including thirty documented benefits of the ketogenic diet outside of weight loss. These benefits were found through scientific research, and many were shared by people who have implemented the ketogenic diet independently. In some cases, the diet was used on its own. In other cases, it was used in coordination with other therapies, which may have included medications while working closely with a medical healthcare professional.

1. Stabilizes energy
2. Regulates hunger
3. Lowers triglycerides
4. Starves cancer cells
5. Stabilizes blood sugar
6. Reduces inflammation
7. Reduces blood pressure
8. Assists in craving control
9. Type 2 diabetes remission
10. Stage 4 cancer remissions
11. Improves hormonal balance
12. Type 1 diabetes management
13. Reduces metabolic syndrome
14. Reduces or eliminates migraines
15. Improves symptoms of Psoriasis
16. Reduces symptoms of ADD/ADHD
17. Traumatic brain injury management
18. Improves or eliminates sleep apnea
19. Decreases several known birth defects
20. Enhances brain function & brain health
21. Decreases PTSD symptoms & episodes
22. Reduces or removes seizures in children
23. Increases "feel good" endorphins & mood
24. Protection against cardiovascular diseases
25. Increases genetic diversity of the gut microbiome
26. Improves endurance (in trained and untrained people)
27. Improves or eliminates non-alcoholic fatty liver disease
28. Decreases symptoms of dementia & Alzheimer's disease
29. Improves symptoms of polycystic ovarian syndrome (PCOS)
30. Reduces psychiatric illness symptoms (Schizophrenia, Bipolar, Depression, Autism, ADHD, OCD)

Even though weight loss is a fantastic bonus for many in this way of life, there are several other incredible benefits to overall health and wellness for many people who have changed over to the ketogenic lifestyle. Not to mention that it makes you feel amazing. So much so that researchers have reported that some study participants refused to stop the diet at a certain point during research studies. According to Dr. Ian Campbell of Edinburgh University, participants refused to stop the diet because they said they felt better than ever. As you can guess, this is challenging for the researchers trying very hard to get their findings and results out to the public.

Hundreds, if not thousands, of studies and trials are being performed on the ketogenic diet daily for many different uses in various areas of health and wellness. At this point, the ketogenic diet has been through enough research and trials, proving that its health benefits outweigh any risks and that if it were a prescription drug, it would already be FDA-approved for public use.

However, since it isn't a prescription drug that can be sold to the public and no money can be made on it by our government, the pharmaceutical companies, or most modern-day medical practices, it is "kept in the back of the closet" as a treatment option. It is often kept from people as an option because many medical professionals don't understand it. They don't know how impactful it can be in improving the catastrophic metabolic illnesses that are currently plaguing not just us here in the US but almost every country in the world.

We are finally entering an inspiring time when researchers, scientists, dieticians, nutritionists, and doctors are starting to come together. They share trials, case studies, and research and are opening up dialogs about how their findings could relate to other areas of health and the medical field. Ketogenic diet advocates are starting multi-million dollar research funds to help fund new research on the diet as well.

Leading Nutritional Ketosis & Ketogenic Diet Experts

It is healthy to question things presented to us and only take some things at face value. I want you to be able to do your research and get it from the top medical and science experts in the field. So, I will list some of these top experts for you here.

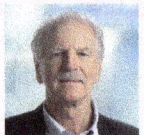

Dr. Stephen D. Phinney, M.D.

Dr. Phinney is a retired Medical Doctor with a Ph.D. in Nutritional Biochemistry and a medical school professor. He is an author and a top lecturer on nutritional ketosis, the ketogenic diet, and low-carb living. Many people call him the "godfather of ketogenic research" as he has studied the diet for over 45 years and practiced it for more than 25 years now. He continues to passionately share his knowledge at several of the world's top low-carb and metabolic conferences. You can learn more about him here:
https://www.virtahealth.com/people/stephen-phinney

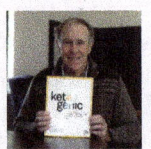

Professor Tim Noakes, Ph.D.

Professor Noakes is a sports scientist and an emeritus professor at the Division of Exercise Science and Sports Medicine at the University of Cape Town. He obtained his medical degree in 1974 and his doctoral degree in 1981, followed by a second doctoral for academic science research in Exercise Science in 2002. He is an avid runner and marathoner. He was a high-carb advocate for several years before admitting publicly that he was wrong. His change in opinion occurred after both he and his father were diagnosed with type 2 diabetes after they both had followed the food guidelines for their entire lives.
You can learn more about him here:
https://thenoakesfoundation.org/prof-tim-noakes/

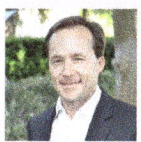

Jeff S. Volek, Ph.D. | RDN

Dr Volek is a Registered Dietician with a Ph.D. in Kinesiology/Nutrition. Dr. Volek is also a top lecturer and professor who runs an Ohio State University (OSU) lab dedicated to studying ketosis, ketones, keto adaptability, and their effects on human metabolism and performance. He is a sought-after presenter and speaker on the ketogenic diet for human performance. You can learn more about him here:
https://ehe.osu.edu/directory?id=volek.1

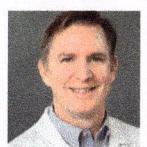

Dr. Eric C Westman, M.D

Dr. Westman is an Internal Medicine, Primary Care Doctor, and Medical Weight Management Specialist. Dr. Westman is also an Associate Professor of Medicine at Duke University and runs an outpatient clinic there. Most of Dr. Westman's clinical research and study involves documenting and improving the effects of medical nutritional therapies, including those on nutritional ketosis. He has a successful YouTube channel where he shares his medical knowledge and practical ketogenic diet applications. You can learn more about him here:
https://www.dukehealth.org/find-doctors-physicians/eric-c-westman-md-mhs

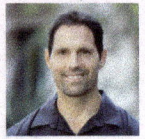

Dominic D'Agostino, Ph.D

Professor D'Agostino has a bachelor's degree in Biological and Nutrition Sciences and a Ph.D. in Physiology and Neuroscience. Dr. D'Agostino is also a top lecturer on the Ketogenic diet, ketones, and exogenous ketones. He runs a lab at the University of South Florida (USF), where they seek to develop and test metabolic-based therapies, such as nutrition and diet, that will improve metabolic health issues. He is the co-founder of a yearly conference, Metabolic Health Summit. He also studies and tests the effects of ketones and exogenous ketones on human brain function. You can learn more about him here:
https://health.usf.edu/medicine/mpp/faculty/ddagosti

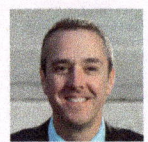

Dr. Chris Palmer, M.D

Dr. Palmer is a practicing psychiatrist at McLean Hospital, Massachusetts General Hospital, and is an Assistant Professor of Psychiatry at Harvard Medical School. He has actively participated in psychiatry and psychiatry research for over 25 years. Dr. Palmer specializes in treatment-resistant mental illness and has been instrumental in the application and use of the ketogenic diet as a form of treatment for psychiatric illnesses in a broad range of disorders. You can learn more about him here:
https://www.chrispalmermd.com/chris-palmer/

There are undoubtedly other leaders in this field. However, only some others have completed the same amount of work these experts have. What they've done and continue to do in studying metabolic syndromes, ketosis, ketones' effects on the human body, and the ability of our body to function optimally with them in our systems is undeniable. Outside of being at the top in their selected fields, they continue seeking more knowledge about ketosis. They find new ways to advance research to improve metabolic health in hopes of helping alleviate the metabolic illness epidemic that the human race is facing.

What's also inspiring is that individuals who have experienced the transformative effects of the ketogenic diet, are joining forces with these healthcare professionals and others like them. They are working together to share their experience through books, podcasts, and social media to inspire and guide others.

The ketogenic diet and lifestyle can do incredible things for your overall mental and physical health, emotional wellness, and longevity. It is about so much more than weight loss!

Next, we will discuss some of the top health challenges we face as a nation before moving on to implementing the ketogenic diet and lifestyle in the last chapters.

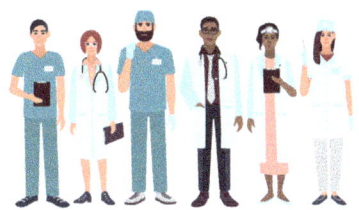

CHAPTER 3: OUR METABOLIC HEALTH CRISIS

I am going to review some data and facts with you in the following few paragraphs concerning being overweight and obese. I do not intend to shame or make anyone feel bad. I seek to provide information and data that is easily accessible in hopes that, as a society, we can all work together and start making some much-needed healthy changes.

It's a known fact in the medical and scientific community that people may not "look" unhealthy from the outside, yet have several internal issues that put them in the class of being metabolically sick and unhealthy. Someone doesn't have to be overweight or obese to be metabolically unhealthy, but those who are have a much greater risk of developing more severe mental and physical health-related issues.

So, what exactly does being overweight or obese mean? The World Health Organization (WHO) provides this definition on its website:

"Overweight is a condition of excessive fat deposits. Obesity is a chronic complex disease defined by excessive fat deposits that can impair health. A body mass index greater than or equal to 25 is overweight, and obesity is a BMI greater than or equal to 30." - WHO

Here are a few other points the WHO lists about being overweight and obese:

- Worldwide adult obesity has more than doubled since 1990, and adolescent obesity has quadrupled.
- In 2022, 1 in 8 people in the world were living with obesity.
- In 2022, 2.5 billion adults (18 years and older) were overweight. Of these, 890 million were living with obesity.
- In 2022, 43% of adults aged 18 years and over were overweight and 16% were living with obesity.
- In 2022, 37 million children under the age of 5 were overweight.
- Over 390 million children and adolescents aged 5–19 years were overweight in 2022, including 160 million who were living with obesity.
- If nothing is done, the global costs of overweight and obesity are predicted to reach US$ 3 trillion per year by 2030 and more than US$ 18 trillion by 2060
- Overweight and obesity, as well as their related noncommunicable diseases, are largely preventable and manageable.

It is clear, based on the current data concerning being overweight or obese, that the world has a significant nutrition and lifestyle problem on its hands. Luckily, diet and lifestyle are controllable factors, and they are things we can take into our own hands and change. This is not to say that it is the only cause of human illness or disease in the world, but out of all the factors, nutrition and lifestyle are the factors we can directly affect.

Leading Causes Of Death In The United States
On the next page is a graph of the top ten leading causes of death in the US for 2022. Of the ten leading causes of death, seven are mainly lifestyle-related and could possibly be pre-

vented. There are hereditary factors as well. I do not want to dismiss this fact. However, our current health state here in the US is progressively getting worse and worse, year over year, and that is not just genetics.

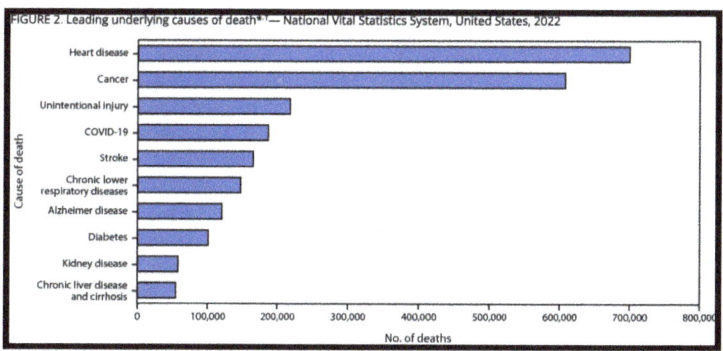

The Centers For Disease Control (CDC) states,

"Heart disease, cancer, diabetes, and stroke are among the most common causes of illness, disability, and death in the United States. They also drive the nation's $4.1 trillion in annual health care costs." **- CDC**

All of these killers can be sufficiently reduced or, in some cases, eliminated with weight reduction and overall metabolic health improvement, which can be achieved with the ketogenic diet and lifestyle.

Heart disease and strokes have been the leading causes of death in the US since the 1920s. That's well over 100 years, and no medical advancements, prescriptions, or diets have helped reduce their rankings on this list. Cancer has been a leading cause of death since the 1930s. This area has better advancements, but it is still number two on the list.

Next up, we have COVID. A very high percentage of the people who got severe COVID or died from it had pre-existing metabolic issues. These issues could have included or been a combination of the following: insulin resistance, being overweight, obese, diabetes, heart issues, lung issues, and inflammation.

Below are statements from the CDC's Obesity, Race/Ethnicity, and COVID-19 paper from their website concerning COVID and its link to being overweight or obese:

Adults with excess weight are at even greater risk during the COVID-19 pandemic:
- Having obesity increases the risk of severe illness from COVID-19. People who are overweight may also be at increased risk.
- Having obesity may triple the risk of hospitalization due to a COVID-19 infection.
- Obesity is linked to impaired immune function.
- Obesity decreases lung capacity and reserve and can make ventilation more difficult.
- More than 900,000 adult COVID-19 hospitalizations occurred in the United States between the beginning of the pandemic and November 18, 2020. Models estimate that 271,800 (30.2%) of these hospitalizations were attributed to obesity.
- A study of COVID-19 cases suggests that risks of hospitalization, intensive care unit admission, invasive mechanical ventilation, and death are higher with increasing BMI.
  - The increased risk for hospitalization or death was particularly pronounced in those under age 65.

Next on the list are Alzheimer's disease and diabetes. Alzheimer's didn't appear on the leading causes of death list until 1994. Diabetes didn't hit the list until the early 2000s. Diabetes was higher on this list until Alzheimer's overtook it in 2007. Today, Alzheimer's disease is referred to by many doctors and medical experts as type 3 diabetes. Having diabetes doubles your risk of getting Alzheimer's.

It's estimated that 38.4 million people have type 2 diabetes. 8.7 million of the 38.4 million have not been diagnosed, and most don't even know they have it. 97.6 million people are pre-diabetics. These are staggering numbers. Approximately 1 in 3 adults with diabetes also have chronic kidney disease, which comes in ninth on the leading causes of death list. Implementation of the ketogenic diet and lifestyle change can reduce these numbers significantly. Drs. Phinney and Volek co-founded Virta Health. The Virta Health medical practice was created to help with this massive diabetes health crisis. Virta Health aims to reverse type 2 diabetes in over 100 million people without medications or surgeries. Reduction in type 2 diabetes will not only reduce deaths from this disease, but it will also reduce deaths from type 3 (Alzheimer's) diabetes.

Lastly, we have liver disease and cirrhosis. For many years, the prevalence of liver disease was primarily associated with alcohol or drugs or one of the three forms of hepatitis. Around the mid-1980s, this started to change with the prevalence of more sugar consumption, weight gain, and type 2 diabetes. Now, overconsumption of carbs and sugar is a leading cause of nonalcoholic fatty liver disease (NAFLD) in younger people, teens, and children as young as three years old. It is estimated that 100 million people in the United States have NAFLD.

While mental illness didn't directly make the list of causes of death, it is an important issue that we face in the US, and it is playing a role in some of the leading causes of death. In 2023, reported depression rates reached a new high. It was reported that 29% of the US population has reported being diagnosed with depression, 10% higher than in 2015, and 17.8% of those are reporting that they are currently depressed. Women have experienced the most significant overall increase, with one-third being diagnosed with depression.

There are significant scientific advancements in the studies of people with mental illnesses. People who have depression, schizophrenia, or bipolar disorders most of their lives are now seeing drastic reductions in all of their symptoms after starting a medically supervised ketogenic nutritional therapy. Many of them are in remission, off several medications, and finally living "normal" lives for the first time.

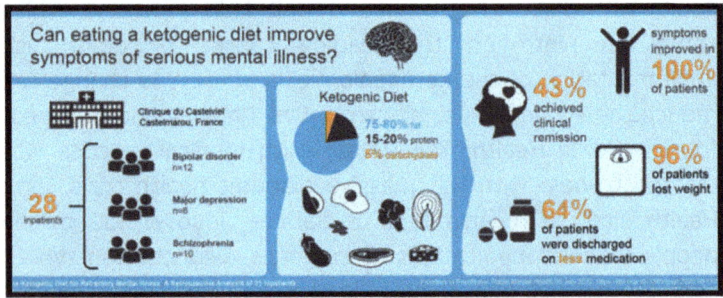

Can you guess what mental illness and all the leading causes of death have in common? You are correct if you guessed the overconsumption of sugar, flour, and carbohydrates.

This isn't just affecting adults. These issues are affecting our kids. If we don't start being the change they need to see, we are sentencing them to a lifelong battle with illnesses, diseases, and possibly even early death. I don't know about you, but I am not okay with that.

Now, let's move on to the basic principles of nutrition and the ketogenic diet so that we can get you started on the path to ketosis.

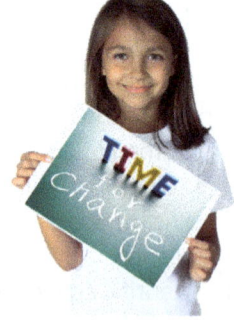

CHAPTER 4: BASIC KETO PRINCIPLES

The basic definition of the ketogenic diet is a diet high in fats, with moderate amounts of protein and minimal carbohydrates.

We are going to talk about macronutrients. Macronutrients (macros) are the nutrients we consume in more significant quantities daily to provide life energy for everyday functioning. We will discuss the three main macronutrients: fats, proteins, and carbohydrates (carbs).

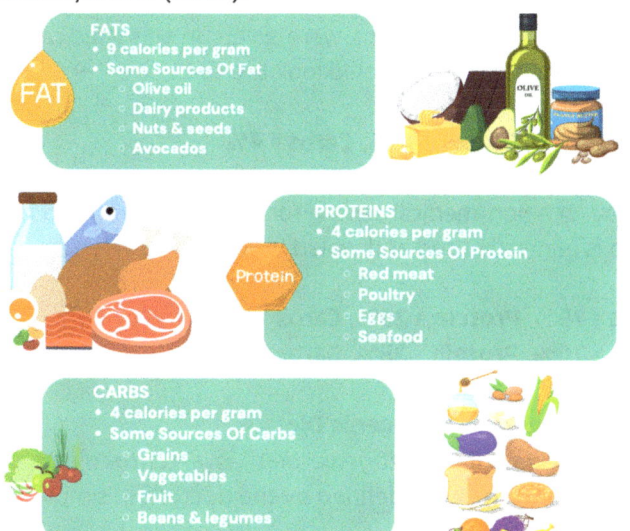

FATS
- 9 calories per gram
- Some Sources Of Fat
  - Olive oil
  - Dairy products
  - Nuts & seeds
  - Avocados

PROTEINS
- 4 calories per gram
- Some Sources Of Protein
  - Red meat
  - Poultry
  - Eggs
  - Seafood

CARBS
- 4 calories per gram
- Some Sources Of Carbs
  - Grains
  - Vegetables
  - Fruit
  - Beans & legumes

While many think all three macros are essential for human survival, only fats and proteins are essential. Let me explain. Carbohydrates turn into glucose in the body, and while glucose is essential, our body can make glucose from protein and fats, making carbs non-essential.

Once consumed, each macronutrient turns into something different in our bodies. When macros are ingested, our digestive system breaks them down as soon as they hit our mouths. The body breaks them down as follows: carbohydrates turn into glucose, proteins become amino acids, and fats (lipids) are broken down into ketones.

Back in the 1920s, when the ketogenic diet was used for children with epilepsy, they established the first dietary recommendation to induce the production of ketones in the body quickly. Dr. Peterman, who worked alongside Dr. Wilder at the Mayo Clinic, suggested that the diet should consist of 1 gram of protein per kilogram of body weight, 10-15 grams of carbohydrates, and the remaining calories should be from fats. This is a 4:1 macronutrient ratio (4 grams of fat per every 1 gram of protein). This was the first time in keto's history that macronutrient breakdowns were given. In this medical setting, that macro breakdown would look like this:

Fats = 90%, Protein = 6%, Carbs = 4%

Today, in a non-medical setting for people like you and me, a 3:1 ratio is generally used and would look like this:

Fats = 75%, Protein = 20%, Carbs = 5%
Fats = 70%, Protein = 25%, Carbs = 5%

Well-Formulated Ketogenic Diet

A *"well-formulated ketogenic diet"* is a term coined by Drs. Phinney and Volek. As defined by the doctors, in simple terms:

Well-Formulated Ketogenic Diet
A diet high in healthy fats, moderate proteins, and minimal carbohydrates, primarily from non-starchy vegetables, with effective electrolyte and mineral management.

Ideally, in a well-formulated ketogenic diet, the carbs would stay between 20 and 25 grams and rarely exceed 50 grams. If your carbs exceed 50 grams, and even lower than 50 for some people, it can prevent the body from making ketones. It would become a low-carbohydrate diet, which still has health benefits but is not ketogenic. There is one exception to this: if someone is an athlete, their carb intake can be higher (50-100 grams), and they can remain in ketosis.

The protein intake should be between 0.7 to 1 gram per pound of ideal body weight, depending on your activity level. If you don't participate in weekly exercise, I suggest you stay on the low end. If you do exercise, I'd recommend staying on the higher end. Ideally, you want to get at least 30 grams of protein (25 grams if from whey protein powder) per meal to activate protein synthesis, an essential component of how our bodies build and maintain muscle mass.

Lastly, fat will be the remainder of your calorie intake. Fat intake should stay between 65% and 80% of your daily calorie consumption.

A well-formulated ketogenic diet should also include a healthy sodium intake. A healthy way to consume sodium is by using salts, not processed foods. Sodium and electrolyte balance are essential because the body, specifically the liver, will process sodium differently once the carbs are lowered. If you don't add enough sodium to your diet, you will feel a lack of energy or even slightly fatigued, which many call "keto flu." Try adding an electrolyte blend or a broth if you are adding sodium from salts and still feeling sluggish.

Nutritional Ketosis

The ketogenic diet aims to have your body run on ketones for your life energy. When your body is running on ketones for fuel instead of glucose, this is called nutritional ketosis. Nutritional ketosis is a metabolic state in which ketones become a vital energy source for the body and brain. This is not to be confused with ketoacidosis, which is severe and can become life-threatening for those with diabetes, mainly those with type 1 diabetes. Below is a representation from Dr. Phinney's slides, which he often uses to visually show the difference between nutritional ketosis and diabetic ketoacidosis.

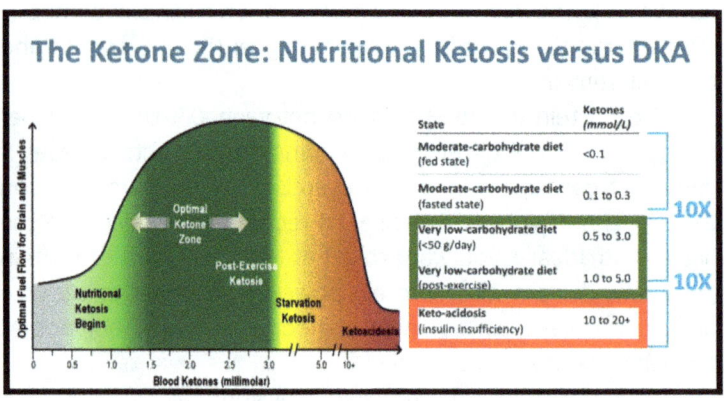

Nutritional ketosis, which is from 0.5 mmol to 5 mmol, and diabetic ketoacidosis (DKA), which is from 10 mmol to 20+ mmol, are very different levels of blood ketones and far apart on the scale. There is much misinformation about it, so I wanted to show you this visual representation of how far apart they are. I do not want you to be scared of that happening to you if you've heard the myth that a ketogenic diet can cause you harm due to this. For simplicity's sake, I will reference nutritional ketosis as ketosis for the remainder of the book.

Getting into ketosis is a process. While some might jump right in, that isn't everyone's path. I don't think it is advisable for everyone, mentally or physically, to jump haphazardly into the macro ratios I listed earlier. It is estimated that most people eat between 225 and 300 grams of carbohydrates daily. Let me ask you a question: If you eat 225 to 300 grams of carbohydrates daily, will dropping to 20 or 25 grams of carbs tomorrow feel good or be sustainable for you? I'm pretty sure we both know the answer.

I know there's a much more manageable, softer way to get yourself into ketosis without going to extremes. Remember, this is a lifestyle change, not a race. This is why some people fail, and the diet becomes undesirable and unsustainable. They jump into it quickly without appropriately planning or preparing themselves physically or mentally for the change. You must remember that your body has been using carbs for fuel almost your entire life. Changing over to using ketones for fuel is going to take some time, and this is known as keto-adaption. In most cases, initial keto-adaptation can take from 2 to 4 weeks. Full keto-adaptation can take anywhere from six months to one year.

So, how do you get started in a non-extreme way? Great question! Chapter 5 will provide the tools you'll need, how to clean out the pantry, what you can eat, some much-needed tips and tricks, and how and when to get into ketosis. Then, the following chapters will tie it all together to help you make the keto lifestyle an enjoyable, sustainable, healthy way of life.

I have written the following three chapters in a question-and-answer format so that you can quickly locate the answers to your questions. I have included a section within the resource section that lists each question with its corresponding page number(s).

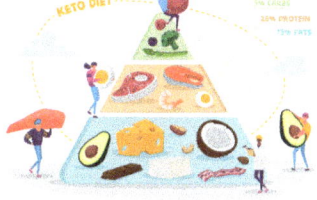

CHAPTER 5: GETTING STARTED

I want to start by giving you some tips on how to set yourself up for success before you start your new ketogenic lifestyle. We will move into commonly asked questions, and I'll wrap up this chapter with guidance on getting into ketosis and what that entails.

How should I clean out my refrigerator and pantry?
When I started this journey, I had all kinds of foodstuff in my refrigerator and pantry that needed to go. I'm not suggesting that you give everything away that doesn't fit this new lifestyle you're embarking on. You do the best you can when you are ready to begin. Even a partial clean-up or clean-out can help get you rolling. While I wish everyone would join this way of life, not everyone will, so there is no need to throw away food when there are people out there who will eat it.

- <u>Unopened/Unused Food – Donate:</u>

Find a local food bank close to your home. Food donation is a great way to give back and help you start this new way of life on the right foot. Get some boxes and start clearing out the canned, boxed, and bagged items you know don't fit your new lifestyle.

- <u>Opened/Partially Used Food - Give Away:</u>

Are you friends with your neighbors? Maybe you can offer them some items you have opened but aren't using any longer. If that's too uncomfortable, ask your family and friends if they want any items.

- <u>Have A Get Together - Use Food You Want To Get Rid Of:</u>

It may have been a while since your favorite friends or family group got together. Use this as an opportunity to cook or use many things you already have while spending quality time with them. This is also a great way to have them see you before the transformation you're about to have. The best part is that when you've improved your health and weight, you can have another get-together to introduce them to the new food you've learned to love. You get to be an example and provide them with much better food than the last get-together you had. Plus, this time, you will look and feel amazing!

I have found a few things that even now, after all this time, I cannot keep in the house because if the right situation arises, I might eat them. I have accepted that and don't bother bringing them into the house. Most, if not all of us, have at least one or a few of those types of foods in our lives. There were other foodstuffs I had to get rid of initially, but after I became fully keto-adapted, they didn't appeal to me as they once did; my cravings for them don't exist anymore.

We've been eating food-like products (boxed and bagged foods) designed to keep us wanting more.

The Bliss Point

The point at which food scientists have found the perfect combination of sugar, fat, salt, and artificial chemicals that will make you want more. Eating these food-like products can cause your body to stop recognizing fullness signals, leading to increased hunger and cravings.

What if I can't clean out my pantry because of other people in my household?

If you know there are things you just will not be able to abstain from if they are in the house, I say get rid of them, period. Explain to others in your household that you need it out of the house for a short time, not forever. If someone isn't cooperative, ask them if they can keep it in an area you will not see during your adaption period. Do what you can to help make this process as easy as possible.

What foods should I buy?

I'm providing lists for each macronutrient, beverages, and an avoid-replacement list. These lists will not include every food and drink out there that is ketogenic friendly, as I do not know them all, nor is there enough space to include them. I am including as many items as possible that will give you variety without being too overwhelming.

HEALTHY FATS

- Ghee
- Butter
- Olive oil
- Avocado oil
- Avocados
- Coconut oil
- Coconut
- Macadamia oil
- MCT oil
- Heavy cream
- Dark chocolate
- Seed butter
- Greek yogurt
- Hard cheeses
- Soft cheeses
- Hemp hearts
- Nuts
- Seeds
- Fatty fish
- Eggs
- Fatty cuts of meat
- Rendered animal fats (lard and tallows)
- Mayo (made from healthy oils, NOT seed oils)

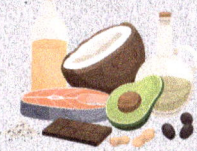

COLORFUL KETO

PROTEINS

Eggs
Red meats
Organ meats
White meats
Seafood
Fish
Cheese
Nuts
Seeds
Tofu
Bone broth
Greek yogurt
Natural sausages
Natural lunch meats
Whey protein isolates

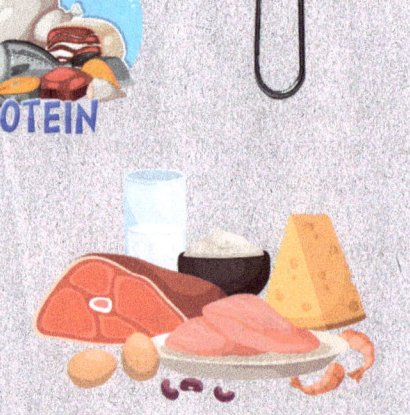

VEGETABLES

Suggested 2 to 3 Servings Per Day:
Asparagus (4 to 8 stalks)
Broccoli (½ to 1 cup)
Cucumbers - Minis (1 to 2)
Brussels Sprouts (6 to 8 sprouts)
Olives (6 to 12 olives)
Spinach & Kale (1 to 2 cups)
Zucchini (½ to 1 cup)
Garlic (½ to 1 tbsp)
Cauliflower (½ to 1 cup)
Green beans (½ to 1 cup)
Radishes (1 to 1½ cups)
Mushrooms (½ to 1 cup)
Onions & Peppers (¼ to ½ cup)
Lettuces (1 to 2 cups; high water content)
Celery (2-4 stalks; high water content)
Cabbage (½ to 1 cup; great pre-biotic fiber)

FRUITS

Suggested 1 to 2 Servings Per Day:
Strawberries (½ of a cup)
Plums – Small (½ to 1)
Clementine (½ to 1)
Blueberries (¼ of a cup)
Cherries (¼ of a cup)
Kiwi – Small (½ to 1)
Cantaloupe (½ of a cup)
Peach – Small (½ to 1)
Lemon/Lime (½ to 1)
Tomatoes – Medium (½ to 1)
Starfruit – (¼ to ½ of a cup)
Coconut – (¼ to ½ of a cup)
Blackberries (¼ a cup, high in fiber)
Raspberries (¼ a cup, high in fiber)
Avocado – Minis (½ to whole mini, high in fiber)

BEVERAGES

Filtered water
Lemon water
Heavy cream
Coffee
Tea
Sparkling water
Soda water
Apple cider vinegar
Tonic water
Bouillon
Bone broths
Nut milk (unsweetened)
Coconut milk (unsweetened)

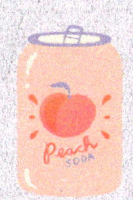

What foods should I avoid? What do I replace them with?

This may seem obvious at first. However, little things can trip you up if you don't know substitutes for everyday food items that you will remove from your diet to make it sustainable and effective. I'm providing you with common foods to avoid on the left side of the list, then replacement suggestions for you on the right. This will be a handy reference list for you in the future, and it makes a great printout to keep in your kitchen or carry with you when you are out and about.

FOODS TO AVOID	REPLACEMENTS
Table Sugar Or Added Sugars	Monk fruit, stevia, xylitol, erythritol, allulose
Regular Pasta	Zucchini, shirataki or palm noodles, konjac flour pasta
White Or Whole Grain Breads	Lettuce, almond flour-based bread
Tortillas	Lettuce, egg wraps, almond or coconut flour-based wraps
Potatoes	Cauliflower, radishes, (also see vegetable list)
All Purpose Flour	Almond, coconut or konjac flour
Beans	Mushrooms, ground meat, (also see protein list)
Rice	Cauliflower, broccoli, konjac or shirataki rice
Margarine, Crisco Or Vegetable Oils	Butter, ghee, avocado oil (high heat) or olive oil (low heat)

GETTING STARTED

FOODS TO AVOID	**REPLACEMENTS**
Half & Half	Heavy cream or unsweetened nut or coconut milk
Regular Milk	Heavy cream or unsweetened nut or coconut milk
Fruit Juices	Homemade fruit-flavored water, stevia sparkling water
Beer	Bud Light Next, Corona Premier, Yuengling Flight
Wine	Dry Farm, Gratsi, FitVine, Palo61, Revel
Mixed Drinks	Use soda water or tonic, lime/lemon & stevia to flavor
Regular Or Diet Sodas	Sparkling, soda, or tonic waters, (also see beverage list)
Milk chocolate	Pure dark chocolate 75% and up
Chips Or Crackers	Almond flour or cauliflower based items, cheese crisps
Oatmeal	Chia seed, hemp or flaxseed puddings
Granola	Chopped nuts and seeds mixed together
Pre-Packaged Trail Mix	Make your own; healthy nuts and homemade dried berries

FOODS TO AVOID	**REPLACEMENTS**
Dried Fruit	Berries, cherries, homemade dried fruits (also see fruit list)
Croutons Or Bread Crumbs	Crushed hard cheese crips or pork rinds
Corn	Cauliflower rice, (also see vegetable list)
Baby Carrots	Celery, broccoli, cauliflower, (see vegetable list)
Bananas	Berries, avocado, (also see fruit list)
Honey	Honey substitutes made with allulose, stevia or monk fruit
Regular Lunch Meats	Lower sodium, nitrate & BHB free meats or cut your own

I would also like to warn you about the marketing masters when shopping for prepackaged food. Just because the package says it's low-carb, keto, or keto-friendly on the front does not mean it is!

When purchasing prepackaged foods, carefully read the nutrition label and ingredients list on the back. You'll want to ensure that there are minimal carbs, minimal to no added sugars, and a limited amount of chemical fillers because they are not good for you. The more pronounceable the ingredients are, the better it will be for you to consume. I have provided a comparison example on the next page to see the difference. Also, please pay attention to the serving size so you don't accidentally overconsume it. Serving sizes are not based on nutritional facts but on average reported consumption.

GETTING STARTED

TERRIBLE

INGREDIENTS: ENRICHED FLOUR (WHEAT FLOUR, NIACIN, REDUCED IRON, THIAMIN MONONITRATE [VITAMIN B₁], RIBOFLAVIN [VITAMIN B₂], FOLIC ACID), CORN SYRUP, SUGAR, SOYBEAN AND PALM OIL (WITH TBHQ FOR FRESHNESS), CORN SYRUP SOLIDS, DEXTROSE, HIGH FRUCTOSE CORN SYRUP, FRUCTOSE, GLYCERIN, CONTAINS 2% OR LESS OF COCOA (PROCESSED WITH ALKALI), POLYDEXTROSE, MODIFIED CORN STARCH, SALT, DRIED CREAM, CALCIUM CARBONATE, CORNSTARCH, LEAVENING (BAKING SODA, SODIUM ACID PYROPHOSPHATE, MONOCALCIUM PHOSPHATE, CALCIUM SULFATE), DISTILLED MONOGLYCERIDES, HYDROGENATED PALM KERNEL OIL, SODIUM STEAROYL LACTYLATE, GELATIN, COLOR ADDED, SOY LECITHIN, DATEM, NATURAL AND ARTIFICIAL FLAVOR, VANILLA EXTRACT, CARNAUBA WAX, XANTHAN GUM, VITAMIN A PALMITATE, YELLOW #5 LAKE, RED #40 LAKE, CARAMEL COLOR, NIACINAMIDE, BLUE #2 LAKE, REDUCED IRON, YELLOW #6 LAKE, PYRIDOXINE HYDROCHLORIDE (VITAMIN B₆), RIBOFLAVIN (VITAMIN B₂), THIAMIN HYDROCHLORIDE (VITAMIN B₁), CITRIC ACID, FOLIC ACID, RED #40, YELLOW #5, YELLOW #6, BLUE #2, BLUE #1.

Whopping 60 ingredients;
(7) types of sugar, (6) types of sodium/preservatives, (3) types of oils (7) food dyes.

GREAT

Organic * Gluten Free
Vegan
Ingredients: Organic Nori, Organic Sunflower Seeds, Organic Macadamia Nuts, Organic Apple Cider Vinegar, Organic Tomato, Organic Lemon, Sea Salt
1.5 oz. ORGANIC contains tree nuts
TreeCafe.co...

Only 8 ingredients;
Organic ingredients, you can pronounce them all.

Your goal should be to eat as much whole-natural food as possible. This is not a request for you to do this 100% of the time because that isn't feasible in our world with the hustle and bustle of everyday life for most of us. Try your best to stay with the 80/20 Rule. Eat as best as possible at least 80% of the time, and then allow yourself some grace for the other 20%. I will discuss food quality and types in Chapter 7.

Should I take any vitamins and/or supplements?

Many people think they don't need supplements and vitamins, while some may take too many. I always say, *"You can't outwork or outsupplement a bad diet."*

There should be a middle ground, not too much or too little, in coordination with your local pharmacists. I say in coordination with your local pharmacists because you want to ensure that any supplements you consider won't interfere with any medications you might be on. Your local pharmacist is the best resource for information on these interactions.

Vitamin Supplement List:
- Sodium (pink Himalayan, sea salt, or ionized salt)
- Magnesium (glycinate, citrate, malate - best absorbed)
- Magnesium + Chloride (optimal for sleep and immunity)

Sodium: While we often hear "salt is bad," it depends on the context. Many times, it isn't the table salt that is the problem. It is the sodium coming from processed foods. If most of your diet comes from processed foods with massive amounts of sodium, this can cause significant issues. However, since our goal on the ketogenic diet is to minimize processed foods, we must get our sodium more naturally and healthily through different types of salts.

We are talking about increasing salt intake because our kidneys process salt differently when we get into ketosis and after becoming keto-adapted. Current research suggests 5 to 8 grams or 5000 to 8000 milligrams daily when practicing the ketogenic diet.

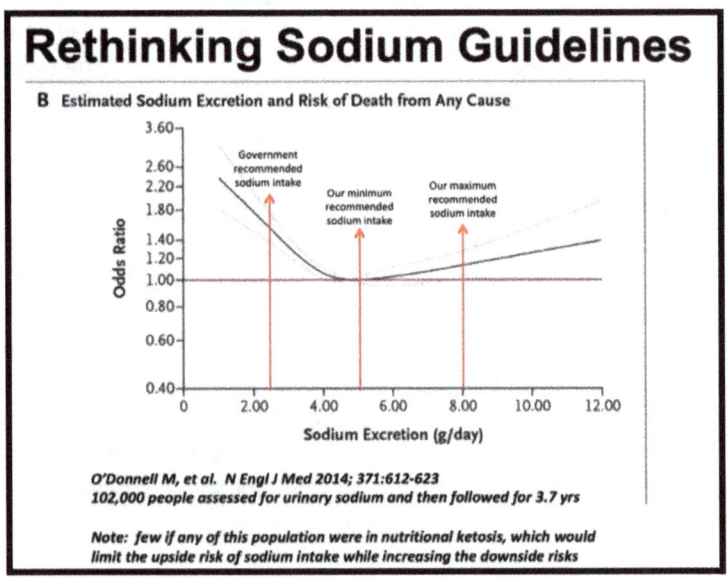

Magnesium: It is used for 300+ different enzymatic processes in the body, and it is essential to your overall health and the optimal ketogenic lifestyle. It is critical for bone health, blood pressure, cardiovascular function, muscle functioning, energy production, regulating blood sugar, and assists with nervous and immunity systems functioning. It has also been shown to enhance mood and reduce stress and anxiety.

Different people experience different effects with certain types of magnesium. I have provided you with various kinds. If you try a particular type and you have symptoms you don't like, switch to another kind that doesn't give you adverse effects. Many people take multiple types to get the maximum health benefits.

Vitamin Supplement List (Cont.):
- Vitamin D3 (K2 helps with the absorption of this)
- Omega 3s OR Omega 3-6-9 Blend (combination of fish and other oils - Best)
- Pro-Biotic w/Pre-Biotic (16 Billion plus strands - Best)

Supplements (Other/Optional) List:
- Electrolytes (sodium, magnesium, potassium with added chloride and calcium - Best)
- Whey protein powder (isolate form - Best)
- Plant-based protein powder (pea protein - Best)
- Turmeric (full spectrum - Best)
- Creatine monohydrate (micronized form - Best)
- Exogenous ketones (see Chapter 7 for more information on these)

What kitchen tools and accessories will I need?
When I first started, I bought various kitchen accessories. I spent too much money and filled my cabinets with things I rarely used or only used once or twice. I don't want you to make the same mistakes that I did or waste your hard-earned money.

On the next page, I will list the items that have made keto life more manageable and food preparation and cooking much quicker. Outside of weekly food prep, I rarely take more than 30 minutes to prep and cook meals these days.

Kitchen - Must Haves:
Glass or metal water bottle
Filtered water
Measuring spoons
Measuring cups
Glass oil sprayers
Basic kitchen shears
Handheld Grater
6-speed handheld mixer
Mini food chopper
Steamer basket
Air-Fryer
Small baking pans
Tongs
Frying pan
Large baking sheet
Cupcake pan
Parchment paper
Tin foil
Baggies
BPA-free storage containers
BPA-free meal prep containers

Kitchen - Optional:
Multi-level steamer
Hard-boiled egg cooker
2-In-1 food cutting shears
Food processor or blender
Instant Pot
Crock Pot
Silicone cooking mats
Countertop mixer
Copper pans
Cast iron pans
Glass storage containers
Glass meal prep containers
Silicone cupcake holders

Will I have to food prep every week?

Everyone's life looks different, so every food prep looks different. The best way is the way that works best for you. Below are a few ideas that may appeal to you.

- Prepare & cook breakfast bits (see resource section)
- Prepare & make lunch or dinner boxes
- Batch* cook meat or veggies (1-3 lb & 1-3 types)
- Cut up fruit & vegetables then portion out
- Baggie marinate meat & freeze (use monthly or weekly)

*Batch cook means cooking large amounts of things simultaneously.

Will I have to track my food?

I understand that many people prefer to avoid tracking their food intake. If you want to change your weight and health, it is necessary for your food to be tracked initially and then periodically for a week here and there later to ensure you are staying on track.

My Fitness Pal is the app I am most familiar with for tracking food. There are several others out there, such as Cronometer and Lose It. Cronometer allows you to keep track of more micronutrients than any other app, making me consider switching, but I have not done so yet. All of these can be found in your phone app store. Feel free to use the one you will be most comfortable using to make it more manageable.

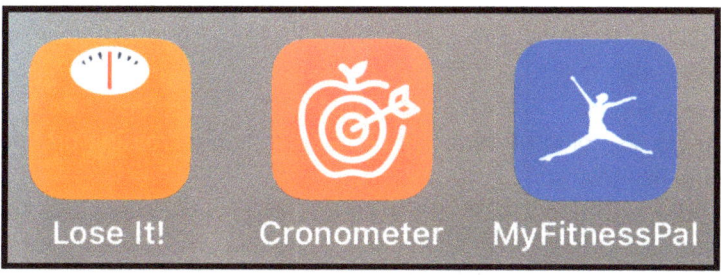

Why should I track my food?

We often need to pay more attention to how much we eat and drink and be aware of how many grams of carbs are hidden in our daily consumption. This can add up quickly and keep us from getting into ketosis or kick us out of ketosis. What we track gets better, and it isn't forever!

How do I get into ketosis?

I will provide three routes to ketosis because everyone's starting point differs. For the first of the three routes, we will start with someone who consumes less than 99 carbs daily and work up from there.

Route 1: 1-Week Roadmap To Ketosis
(Suggested for those consuming <99 carbs daily)

Week 1: We are ready to implement the first ketogenic macronutrient profile, increase healthy fats, and decrease carbs to a ketogenic level. Choose one of the following:
- Fats = 70%, Protein = 25%, Carbs = 20 to 25 grams
- Fats = 75%, Protein = 20%, Carbs = 20 to 25 grams

Route 2: 3-Week Roadmap To Ketosis
(Suggested for those consuming 100 to 199 carbs daily)

Week 1: Reduce carb intake, increase protein, and increase healthy fats.
Reduce carbs by 35%. Set a Week 1 daily carb intake goal for yourself.
- Fats = 55%, Protein = 25%, Carbs = 20%

Week 2: Continue reducing carb intake and increasing protein and healthy fats.
Reduce carbs by 40%. Set a Week 2 daily carb intake goal for yourself.
- Fats = 65%, Protein = 25%, Carbs = 10%

Week 3: We are ready to implement the first ketogenic macronutrient profile, increase healthy fats, and decrease carbs to a ketogenic level. Choose one of the following:
- Fats = 70%, Protein = 25%, Carbs = 20-25 grams
- Fats = 75%, Protein = 20%, Carbs = 20-25 grams

The first two routes to ketosis will happen within 1 to 3 weeks since the carb intake was lower than average. The initial adaptation period will cause some discomfort; the goal is to minimize that as much as possible so the final route will take 5 weeks.

GETTING STARTED

Route 3: 5-Week Roadmap To Ketosis
(Suggested for those currently consuming 200< carbs daily)

Week 1: Reduce carb intake and increase protein to help reduce hunger.
Reduce carbs by 20%. Set a Week 1 daily carb intake goal for yourself.
Week 2: Continue reducing carbs and increasing protein to help reduce hunger.
Reduce carbs by 25%. Set a Week 2 daily carb intake goal for yourself.
Week 3: Continue reducing carbs and increasing protein to help reduce hunger.
Reduce carbs by 30%. Set a Week 3 daily carb intake goal for yourself.
Week 4: We are ready to implement the first ketogenic macronutrient profile, increase healthy fats, and decrease carbs to a ketogenic level.
- Fats = 65%, Protein = 25%, Carbs = 10%

Week 5: We are ready to implement the second ketogenic macronutrient profile, increase healthy fats, and decrease carbs to a ketogenic level. Choose one of the following:
- Fats = 70%, Protein = 25%, Carbs = 20-25 grams
- Fats = 75%, Protein = 20%, Carbs = 20-25 grams

I have provided three ways to get into ketosis based on your current carbohydrate consumption. You are encouraged to use the path that best fits your carbohydrate consumption. However, if you are ready to get into ketosis sooner rather than later and use one of the first routes, I would like to let you know in advance that your fatigue is likely to be worse. It might be rough physically and mentally, so please be aware.

CARB NOTE: To get into ketosis quickly, you will initially want to keep your carbs as low as possible. After you fully detox your body from the carbs, you can adjust the total grams of carbs per day. To get this lifestyle's most optimal health and wellness benefits, you will want to stay under 50 grams of carbs.

PROTEIN NOTE: Staying between 0.7 and 1 gram per lb of your ideal weight is sufficient to promote quicker results. You cannot lose fat without also losing some muscle mass. Your goal should be to prevent muscle loss as much as possible by keeping your daily protein intake sufficient. I suggest you keep your protein from getting higher than 1 gram per lb of your ideal weight initially because it may keep you from getting into ketosis.

FAT NOTE: It takes time for the body to shift from a carb burner to a fat burner. Your body has been using carbs for energy for years, and it will take months to fully adapt to being a fat burner. Some people are more satiated consuming 25% protein and 70% fats, while 20% protein and 75% fat work better for others. If the fat ratio you picked doesn't keep your hunger at bay after two weeks, try the other. I will discuss what to do for prolonged cravings in Chapter 6.

How do I calculate my calories?

There are hand calculation methods, or you can utilize one of the two online sources I have provided below. I suggest that females never go below 1300 calories and males below 1600.

SIMPLE HAND CALCULATION:
Your ideal body weight x 12 (Not Active)
Your ideal body weight x 14 (Semi-Active)
Your ideal body weight x 16 (Very Active)

ONLINE CALCULATORS:
https://tdeecalculator.net/
https://www.calculator.net/calorie-calculator.html

How do I calculate my specific macronutrients?

The easiest way to do this is within your food-tracking app after you have calculated your total daily calories. However, if you aren't using an app, you must use the calculations I provided. Below is an example of the math you'd use to determine your daily ranges for the three macronutrients. For this example, we will use 1800 calories daily with a 20-carb-per-day limit.

Example Daily Calories = 1800 calories

References: Carbs = 4 cal/gram | Fats = 9 cal/gram | Proteins = 4 cal/gram

- Carbs = 20 grams (20x4) = 80 calories; Now, we subtract the 80 calories from 1800, leaving us with 1720 calories.
- Remaining Calories = 1720
- Fats = 75% (1720 x .75) = (1290/9) = 143.33 grams
- Proteins = 20% (1720 x .20) = (344/4) = 86 grams

Total Daily Macros: Carbs = 80 | Fats = 144 | Protein = 86 grams

How flexible can I be with this diet?

To get into ketosis quickly, you will want to be strict at first and stick to 20 to 25 grams of carbs per day. It isn't forever, I promise! Sometimes, you have to get strict again later in the process for short periods. It is all part of living a ketogenic lifestyle. Being strict with your food 30 to 90 days a year to live a healthy, happy life isn't a bad deal. There are more challenging things to deal with, such as being overweight and energy less, heart disease, stroke, cancer, diabetes, Alzheimer's, and other metabolic diseases. As a good friend of mine likes to say, *"You get to choose your hard."*

You may be able to be a little more flexible later, and you may not. We are all different in this aspect, and there is no one-size-fits-all. If your weight, energy levels, sleep, and overall health markers are within healthy ranges and you feel good, stick with what works.

One of the many beautiful benefits of the ketogenic lifestyle is that you don't always have to be in ketosis, nor will you be naturally. Sometimes, your body will naturally slip out of ketosis (see next questions for more specifics on this). This is all part of the process. We may make changes that induce the need for macro changes to continue getting the optimal health benefits that we seek. I will talk more about this in Chapter 7.

How will I know if I am in ketosis?

There are several ways to know if you are in ketosis. The way you feel will be your first sign. Consider testing in the initial stages so that you can associate the better feelings with levels of ketosis in your body. Getting in tune with your body is essential because different ketosis ranges have different feelings. You should be aware of those feelings so that later, when you aren't testing, you will know when you aren't regularly in ketosis so that you can make adjustments accordingly. I'll go over the four ways so that you can better understand each and decide what works best for you.

Feelings (Not in any specific order):

- Sense of clarity and focus enhanced
- Productivity levels increase
- More energy throughout the day
- Reduction in sugar cravings
- Reduction in overall hunger
- Hangry feelings go away
- Fat loss happening
- Wanting to move your body more
- Sleeping for more extended periods
- Feeling more rested when you wake up

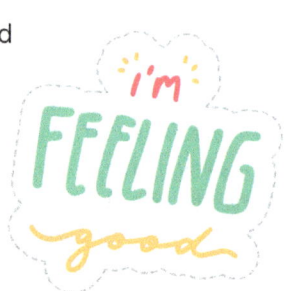

Urine Testing:

Urine testing is only good at the beginning of your journey (first 1 to 3 weeks) because your body isn't using all the ketones it is making yet. These are test strips that you pee on, and they are relatively cheap, usually ranging from $10 to $30. The ones on the higher end typically test for other health markers, not just ketones. As you progress into being a fat burner (your body is running on ketones instead of glucose), there will be fewer ketones in your urine because your body will use them for energy. So, your urine readings won't show accurate ketone levels after a few weeks.

Breathe Testing:
While this method has become popular with some people, it isn't very accurate. It only measures breath acetone, a waste by-product that we breathe out when we are in ketosis. It isn't measuring ketones that the body is producing. However, if you want to know that you are in ketosis, this can be a great option. The price range on these is $50 to $150. The ones on the higher end tend to come with a phone app so that you can keep track of your readings electronically.

Blood Testing:
The fourth and final way is the blood test. It is by far the most accurate way to test the ketone levels in your body. Initial costs are $30 to $60, and ongoing fees can range anywhere from $30 to $50 per month, depending on how frequently you test. The main drawback is that you must prick your finger to get the blood readings. While someone might already be accustomed to this, it can become cumbersome for those who haven't had to do this regularly.

What should my ketone readings be like?
The human body is a magnificent machine, and we have internal individuality, so there isn't always a correct answer regarding what your specific ketones should be reading. As discussed, the nutritional ketosis range is between 0.5 mmol and 5 mmol when measuring your blood ketones. As long as you are staying above

0.5 mmol, then you are in ketosis. You will not be in ketosis 24/7, generally speaking. Some examples of times you might not be in ketosis include morning glucose spikes, post-workout, over your carbohydrate threshold, high stress, or times of sickness. Usually, your numbers will return within a few hours or a few days, depending on why the ketosis stopped.

What will my plate look like?

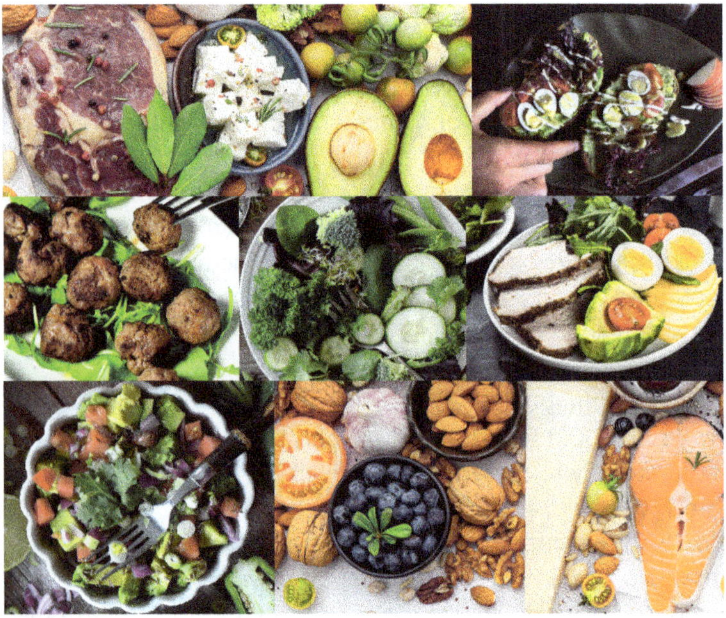

It's pretty colorful food. Keto doesn't have to be dull or colorless. Every time I mention to someone that I live a ketogenic lifestyle that doesn't practice this way of life, without fail, they usually say something like, *"So that's lots of cream cheese and bacon, right?"* Of course, I laugh every time and then respond by saying, *"Those things do make everything better, but it is so much more than that!"*

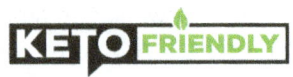

CHAPTER 6: NAVIGATING CHALLENGES

We got you through the first part of this beautiful journey. You know how to prepare, what to eat, some beginning tips, and how to get into ketosis. Now, we will talk about some snags you could run into or challenges you might face as you progress through keto-adaptation. There will be things that come up along the way that you will need some help with. I can't think of every question you might have, but I am confident that I can get through most of the major challenges that will come up.

What is "keto-flu"?
Keto-flu is your body detoxing and withdrawing from excessive carbohydrates and sodium depletion. It was named keto-flu because it exhibits flu-like symptoms such as body aches, lack of energy, fatigue, sugar cravings, nausea, constipation, trouble sleeping, and headaches. Not everyone will experience all of these. Below are some things you can do to help minimize or even eliminate these symptoms.

- Drink plenty of water; increasing water intake to at least half your body weight is suggested.
- Use pink Himalayan or sea salt in the morning (5 to 10 twists/16 oz of liquid); increasing sodium at onset is vital!

- Drink magnesium chloride (helps with electrolyte balance, improves immunity, and promotes relaxation and sleep)
- Use an electrolyte blend (helps with electrolyte balance)
- Broths (bouillon or bone; helps with electrolyte balance)

I'm having problems sleeping, what should I do?

This is very common at first. Many people have issues with their sleep due to the carbohydrate withdrawal process. This doesn't last very long, usually a few days to a week, after shifting into 20 to 25 grams of carbs. Starting a nightly bedtime routine 1 to 2 hours before bed that includes relaxation techniques such as meditation, static stretching, and taking magnesium can help.

What do I do if I have severe food cravings?

If you have severe food cravings, which can be expected for some people, you can bump up your ketogenic ratios to the following: Fats = 80%, Protein = 15%, and Carbs = 20 to 25 grams to help with that. Once your cravings have leveled out, I suggest you return to a lower fat ratio that works best for you. This will take some experimentation until you find the best one for you.

I'm lactose intolerant; do you have suggestions for me?

In my experience, not everyone who is told that they are lactose intolerant is. Often, they have an intolerance to milk due to the amount of lactose plus the added sugar in it, but not to other dairy types with lower lactose and no added sugars, such as butter, cheeses, whey proteins, and creams.

I suggest you implement small amounts of these other dairy options and work your way up. In most cases, you should only consume 1 to 2 oz of these things at a time. I suggest trying ½ to 1 tablespoon of heavy cream at a time to see how you tolerate that. You may find some things you are okay with and others you are not, but you won't know unless you try.

If you try these things and you have issues or you know that you are fully lactose intolerant, there are other options for you to get in healthy fats. You can replace butter with ghee, healthy oils, lard, or tallows. You can replace heavy cream with lactose-free alternatives or powdered versions that you can mix with water that has had the lactose removed. Lastly, you can replace cheeses with dairy-free alternatives from tofu or nuts. Please be careful about the carbohydrate content in the tofu and nut replacements.

If the scale isn't moving, how do I know it's working?

The thing about keto is that only some people lose weight fast. For others, it takes a few weeks or even months. I have for you below the non-scale victories I would like to remind you of.

- Increased energy (after keto-flu)
- More mental clarity and sharpness
- Clothes fit better, looser
- Lose in inches (around total body)
- Sleep quality improves

If you aren't seeing the scale move or experiencing non-scale victories, I suggest you look at your overall calorie intake. Refer back to the section on calculating your daily calorie intake. You might also need to adjust your macro percentages to induce the results you want to achieve.

I'm not getting into ketosis; what should I do?

I will provide a list of the things you need to check that may be causing the issue.

Check Your Macros

- Carb: 20 to 25 grams (MAX for first 3 to 6 months)
- Protein: 0.7 to 0.9 grams per lb of ideal body weight if you don't exercise and no more than 1 gram per lb if you exercise several hours per week.
- Fat: 65 to 80% of your daily calories and ensure you are

Check Your Macros (continued)
- consuming a variety of fats. Examples: healthy oils, heavy cream, fatty meat, nuts, butter, ghee, avocadoes, cream cheese, hard cheese, and seeds

Check Your Stress Levels
- If you are a 7 or above on a scale from 1 to 10 for stress, please implement de-stressing techniques such as walking, exercise, meditation, yoga, reading, quiet time, and a gratitude practice.

If you have checked these things above and after a few weeks you are still not in ketosis, then I would advise that you seek out a ketogenic-friendly professional who can help you figure out what is going on and why this isn't working for you. They can help you find the solution that best fits your needs. Check out the resource section for more information.

What do I do if I slip up or fall off the wagon?
It's not so much if you will fail; it is when. This does not mean that you are a failure. Making life changes is hard. If it were easy, everyone would do it. When you fail, you can get back up and back on track. Don't be afraid to find support if you have difficulty getting back to it. It's OK, we all need a little help sometimes. Please look at the resource section for suggestions.

After you have lived the ketogenic lifestyle for a while, trust me when I say it does get easier. You will want to get back to it sooner rather than later because you will know how good you feel physically and mentally. Remember, this is about your health and longevity, not just weight loss.

I'm constipated; is this normal?
First, let's define constipation and what it is and isn't. Constipation is when you haven't gone poop for days, and you have cramping, pains, nausea, and stomach aches that accom-

pany that. Most of the information you find online is for a Standard American or plant-based diet, which isn't accurate for the ketogenic lifestyle.

When you start fueling your body with more whole-natural foods, you have much less waste to rid the body of. Poop is waste, so you will produce less poop because there will be less waste. As long as less frequent poops are not accompanied by stomach aches, cramps, pain, bloating, or nausea, you should be good to go. Once your body gets keto-adapted, things will naturally straighten out, and you will have a new regularity.

If your issue persists over a few days, try eating walnuts, broccoli, macadamia nuts, or radishes to help move things along. If that doesn't work and you are experiencing discomfort, a last resort would be a magnesium-citrate liquid drink, but make sure you are at home for this one. Any further advice you will need to get from your physician or local pharmacist.

How many meals should I eat per day?
This will be a personal preference. No individual is the same. With my background in nutrition, I always advise my clients to eat between two and four (max) meals per day set within a specific timeframe or an eating window (more on this in Chapter 7).

Can I snack?
First off, snacking isn't a normal human thing. The food manufacturing companies created this to increase sales. Secondly, snacking isn't something you will find very useful once you embrace this way of life because when you fuel your body correctly with ketogenic foods, your hunger level decreases. However, some people accustomed to grazing throughout the day before starting this way of life may find it a little tricky to break this habit right away. It is a mental thing just as much as a physical one.

If you are a snacker or grazer, your weekly goal should be to condense all your food into the number of meals you have decided will work best for you. Be mindful of your snacking because too many snacks can inhibit you from fully getting into ketosis, especially if the snacking is from processed foods.

I've heard my cholesterol might get high; should I be worried?

I am not a doctor or a medical professional; this is not medical advice. The cholesterol story you think you know has been disproven several times since the 1970s. It is not mainstream, and the pharmaceutical companies wouldn't make billions of dollars off high cholesterol (statin) medications each year if it were.

My cholesterol stays between 245 and 285. I know of some people who have even higher cholesterol numbers and still exhibit excellent health and blood work. I suggest you pay attention to your cholesterol and other health markers, not just your blood work. If your doctor doesn't offer you additional options for testing, such as CAC or CCTA scans, and is insistent that you go on statin medications, I strongly advise you to find a new doctor. Seek out a functional or integrative medicine doctor who's a keto-friendly healthcare professional to ensure you stay on the right track for optimal metabolic health. I'll end with a quote from Dr. Charles G Heyd, 1936-1937 president of the American Medical Association:

"For without critical analysis, a doctor would be forever following false leads, leading to no established position in medical practice." **- Charles Heyd**

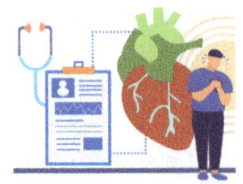

CHAPTER 7: EMBRACING THE KETOGENIC LIFESTYLE

Yay, you've made it to the last chapter, embracing the lifelong journey of the ketogenic diet and lifestyle. Here, I want to quickly review a few things that will make your lifelong journey a little easier and explain some things often discussed in association with the ketogenic lifestyle.

What are "net carbs"?
The term "net carbs" emerged from Dr. Adkins in the 2000s. He later implemented this into his weight loss diet instructions. Net carbs are the total carbs minus any fibers or sugar alcohols you consume. Some argue that you shouldn't count fibers or sugar alcohols because you don't digest them, and they don't affect your blood sugar.

I suggest sticking with total carbs at first to detox your brain and body off carbs and sugar, which is essential to getting into nutritional ketosis. After six months to a year, once you know your carb tolerance and have a solid ketogenic lifestyle built for yourself, experiment with net carbs if you like.

What exactly are MCTs?
MCT stands for medium-chain triglyceride. MCTs are types of fatty acids that are found in high concentrations within coconut

oil. They can also be found in palm kernel oil, but those are not suggested. They help reduce blood sugar, give you brain energy, support weight loss, are known to induce mild states of ketosis, and help you achieve ketosis faster. Some people report mild stomach upset, so it is best to start with ½ a tablespoon and work your way up from there.

What are exogenous ketones?

Exogenous ketones are supplements created to assist people with quickly entering ketosis. Please don't confuse this with being ketogenic. People who elevate their blood ketones with this supplement are not ketogenic, even though they are in ketosis. This means your body isn't producing the ketones; you supplement with external ketones to enter ketosis.

Exogenous ketones only have a temporary effect, usually for a few hours. If taken in correlation with being ketogenic, they can then have additional benefits such as increased energy and focus. If you carb cycle, they can help you get back into ketosis quickly. There are multiple forms: salts, esters, oils, and powders. If you implement these into your diet, purchase only from reputable science-verified manufacturers. I will provide you with a few companies in the resource section.

Will I be able to take breaks?

I don't advise this as a regular practice when you are first starting. If you are a person whose body is highly addicted to carbohydrates, I strongly advise you to stay the course. It is essential to allow your body and your brain time to fully adapt before taking extended breaks. Fully keto-adapted is after someone has been living this way for at least six months to one year.

Another key point is that you won't feel very good or get the most beneficial benefits from this way of life if you are bouncing back and forth. It is important to stay as consistent as possible especially during the beginning stages. The longer you practice this way of life, the more inclined you'll be to stay in ketosis.

VACATIONS OR HOLIDAYS: Some people choose to come off the ketogenic diet entirely during a vacation or holiday when their regular food isn't as readily available. However, I strongly recommend sticking with your regular food as much as possible, even if you aren't entirely in ketosis. Once the vacation or holiday ends, it's important to start back immediately. Avoid getting stuck in old habits for too long, as it can be detrimental to your ketogenic lifestyle.

I've heard about fasting; should I be doing that too?

When it comes to the ketogenic lifestyle, it's best to take things one step at a time. I suggest you focus on the ketogenic diet and lifestyle first before considering other tools. This sequential approach can help you avoid feeling overwhelmed and increase your chances of success.

An eating window would be a better place to start. Having an eating window means you have a set time each day you start eating and a set time to finish eating. For instance, my first solid food meal is around 9:30 a.m. I have my last meal by 7:30 p.m., so I have a 10-hour eating window.

Fasting can be a wonderfully helpful tool physically, mentally, and spiritually that you can implement later down the road once you get fully keto-adapted. Prolonged fasts can enhance your ketone production for the fasting period, but as you refuel your body, the ketone production will slow back down to normal levels.

Are there other keto variations that I can use?

Yes, there are other ratios that can be implemented. You should use the base ratios I provided to fully detox your body from before considering any other ratios unless you have issues. Issues could be digestive or anything where you aren't feeling good after the initial adaption phase (usually 2 to 3 weeks). If you are highly active or work out for several hours per week you may need an adjustment. I will provide some other ratios and methods in the resource section.

What can I eat when out with friends or family?
I suggest you avoid going out to eat for at least the first 30 days to become more quickly keto-adapted and build a solid base of ketone production in your body. If there is a gathering that you cannot miss due to obligation, then I have a few suggestions for you.

1. **Eat a meal before you go.** When you get there, you will be full, which will help prevent you from having something you shouldn't. You can order something light, like a small salad or meat-based appetizer as your entree.
2. **Bring your meal with you.** This way, you can still enjoy the company of your family and friends without deviating from your chosen plan.
3. **Bring diet staples with you.** It is much easier to get your protein and a small salad when you are out; the healthy fats are what usually cause the challenge. Some good examples of things to bring might be your keto dinner rolls, oils you prefer, ghee, nuts, seeds, and dressings.

Can I drink alcohol while living this way?
If you are reading this, I will assume that you are an adult. Alcohol isn't advisable as a regular thing because it is literally a toxin for the body and the mind. Once consumed, your body will immediately process it over everything else, which could lead to a lack of proper nutrient absorption and an overproduction of insulin that can cause the body to store fat instead of burning it for fuel. If you do partake, you can expect a worse hangover, so please proceed with caution. Refer to the avoid/replacements list in Chapter 5 and the reference section for websites with keto-friendly options.

Does the quality or type of meat & eggs I buy matter?

USDA Organic, grass-fed, grass-finished meat or wild-caught fish and seafood are the best options for animal-based items. Purchasing meat that is at least grass-fed is better than the base grocery store's meat. USDA Organic is the best for other foods, such as vegetables and fruits. Eggs are an exception; they are best pasture-raised, as organic means little.

Some labels you see cause a price increase when they do not mean anything about the quality of the product compared to the base level. For instance, if a carton of eggs says that the chicken was fed an all-organic vegetarian diet, please understand that this is not a typical chicken diet. They are omnivores like us and eat grass, seeds, bugs, and worms, not corn, soy, and grains.

If, for budgetary reasons, you cannot afford to get everything in its top quality as listed, start where you can. It's about making small changes you can, as you are able, and not stressing out about it. Once you adapt to this way of life, you will realize you eat much less food volume-wise than before, and making healthier product choices becomes more manageable on your wallet the longer you stick with it.

Grocery Store Base (No Labels):

Animals and fish were fed pumped-up soy, corn, and other grains and raised in poor living conditions. Fruits and vegetables were sprayed with all kinds of chemicals and pesticides that were absorbed into them. When you and I eat these things, we will absorb what these things ate and absorbed before they got to us—just something to think about.

BASE Label Meanings:

Cage Free - chickens were housed and raised together inside a barn but without cages.

Free Range - chickens had "access" to the outdoors, usually something like a small fenced area, but it doesn't necessarily means they have to go outdoors, so be careful here if there aren't more details about whether the animal could roam freely on a farm.

Farm Raised - thousands of fish/seafood kept in a tiny body of water at a time and fed with human-made fish feed (combo of soy, corn, and grains) instead of their natural fish diet.

Vegetarian Feed - you mostly see this on chicken, but it is also popping up on pork, which means the animal wasn't in a natural habitat and was not pasture-raised. Chickens and pigs are omnivores.

BETTER Label Meanings:

Grass-fed - animals were grass-fed until the last three months of their lives, then fed pumped-up soy, corn, and other grains to fatten them.

Non-GMO - was produced without being genetically engineered, and its ingredients weren't derived from genetically modified organisms.

Made With Organic Ingredients - contains at least 70% certified organic ingredients.

BEST Label Meanings:

USDA 100% Organic - 100% produced without chemicals, pesticides, or artificial agents.

USDA Organic - 95% produced without chemicals, pesticides, or artificial agents.

Grass-fed & Grass-finished - animals in a natural habitat where they ate their regular animal diet.

Wild Caught - fish/seafood were caught in a wild habitat, where they ate their regular fish diet.

Pastured Raised - animals were allowed to live freely in a natural habitat, where they ate their regular animal diet.

Do I need to buy all organic vegetables and fruits?
No, you don't need to buy everything organic, but there are

some things you will definitely want to be organic. Every year, a non-profit organization called The Environmental Working Group (EWG) publishes two lists of fruits and vegetables on their website https://www.ewg.org/.

One list is called the Dirty Dozen and includes the fruits and veggies that have the most chemicals and pesticides when tested. The second list is called the Clean Fifteen, and it includes the top fifteen with the least amount of chemicals and pesticides present when they were tested. I am providing you with this list to help you make informed decisions on which you can purchase regular versions of and which are better purchased as organic. NOTE: This list isn't keto-specific.

EWG's 2024 Clean 15 List:	**EWG's 2023 Dirty Dozen List:**
1. Avocados	1. Strawberries
2. Sweet Corn	2. Spinach
3. Pineapples	3. Kale, Collard & Mustard Greens
4. Onions	4. Grapes
5. Papayas	5. Peaches
6. Sweet Peas (frozen)	6. Pears
7. Asparagus	7. Nectarines
8. Honeydew Melons	8. Apples
9. Kiwi	9. Bell & Hot Peppers
10. Cabbage	10. Cherries
11. Watermelon	11. Blueberries
12. Mushrooms	12. Green Beans
13. Mangos	
14. Sweet Potatoes	
15. Carrots	

Will I have to work out to make this work for me?

The diet will work on its own without exercise. That being said exercise is just as important as nutrition and diet. If your goal is to be optimally healthy, then you will definitely want to include exercise. Every step counts, even the tiny baby steps.

Non-Exercisers: After your initial adaption phase or even during it, I suggest you start by taking three dedicated walks a week for 15 minutes if you feel up to it. Once that becomes a habit, increase the length of your walk, and then maybe add some bodyweight exercises before or after your walk and let things naturally progress from there.

Current Exercisers: If you are already working out, I strongly suggest doing very light training sessions for the first two weeks, then progressively increasing until you are adapted. I suggest you do a dedicated walk thrice weekly for about 25 minutes.

Can I build muscle on the ketogenic diet?

Yes, you can! So much conflicting information exists in this area. Many carb-eating bodybuilders will say no, you can't, but this is because they have never actually been fat-adapted. Just getting into ketosis does not make you fat-adapted.

I have been living this lifestyle for over four years and bodybuilding for two years. I have to adjust my macros from time to time to continue the ketogenic lifestyle while building muscle, and I know that it is possible! If you're still unsure, feel free to look up Robert Sikes. He is a 10-year-plus natural ketogenic bodybuilder and is a shining example of the amount of muscle that can be built by eating a ketogenic diet.

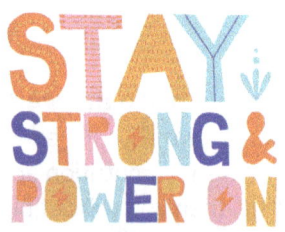

CONCLUSION

"As to disease, make a habit of two things -- To help, or at least, to do no harm."
- Hippocrates

So there you have it, everything that I can think of that will help you start this health-changing and sometimes life-saving ketogenic lifestyle. The science and research being conducted on this diet is amazing. It continues to blow my mind that a simple diet change can impact the human body from deep in the brain to the bottom of our feet. Granted, it is not a one-size-fits-all or a miracle "cure" for everything that affects us. However, it can significantly impact many's health, life, and longevity.

You don't always have to be in ketosis to get the incredible health benefits that this way of life can provide. Many people, including myself, decide to stay on the diet because the mental, physical, and emotional benefits are astounding. There is no desire to change to another way when you enjoy how you feel and what you eat every day. Others practice the diet for months or years and then shift to a different keto variation or lower-carb living. The best way for each individual is the way that best suits their life, which they will stick with, and that keeps them healthy, happy, and well.

The questions I think we should all be asking ourselves is if the ketogenic diet can be so powerful for our health that it has cured epilepsy in some children, reversed type 2 diabetes, put several forms of stage 4 cancers in remission, helped hundreds of other illnesses, and put others in remission; why aren't we hearing more about it at the doctor's office? Secondly, if something as simple as a diet change can help any disease or illness, why is it so vilified and misrepresented by our medical system? Lastly, why do people needlessly suffer because it isn't an approved form of therapy when it's been proven to work in millions of people for over 234 years?

These questions are another reason I felt compelled to write this book. Medical professionals are not really being taught about nutrition. If healthcare professionals took the initiative to educate themselves about nutritional theories independently, it could help to improve the obesity and metabolic health epidemic. Still, nutrition should be a part of basic medical training. Our healthcare system has been functioning as a sick care system, which needs to change. The habit of recommending "eat less and move more" before reaching for the prescription pad is inadequate. Patients should be informed about all available options, not just prescription drugs. It's time that we start using our daily nutrition as a first line of defense against metabolic illness so that we can thrive instead of barely surviving.

I genuinely hope you have enjoyed this book and now have a much better understanding of the ketogenic way of life and the many long-term health and wellness benefits that can make it sustainable.

I am deeply grateful for your time and attention. Your interest in this book is a testament to your commitment to improving your health and wellness. May you experience the transformative power of the ketogenic high that will change your mind and your life, too!

RESOURCES CONTENTS

KETO QUESTIONS AND ANSWERS INDEX
69

OTHER KETOGENIC VARIATIONS
71

EXAMPLE DAILY MEAL PLANS
73

QUICK & EASY KETO RECIPES
77

OTHER RESOURCES
83

REFERENCES
85

KETO QUESTIONS AND ANSWERS INDEX

CHAPTER 5: GETTING STARTED	**PG#**
How should I clean out my refrigerator and pantry?	29-30
What if I can't clean out my pantry?	31
What foods should I buy?	31-33
What foods should I avoid? (Includes replacements)	34-37
Should I take any vitamins and/or supplements?	37-39
What kitchen tools and accessories will I need?	39-40
Will I have to food prep every week?	40
Will I have to track my food?	41
Why should I track my food?	41
How do I get into Ketosis?	41-44
How do I calculate my calories?	44
How do I calculate my specific macronutrients?	45
How flexible can I be with this diet?	45-46
How will I know if I am in ketosis?	46-47
What should my ketone readings be like?	47-48
What will my plate look like?	48

CHAPTER 6: NAVIGATING CHALLENGES	**PG#**
What is "keto flu"?	49-50
I'm having problems sleeping, what should I do?	50
What do I do if I have severe food cravings?	50

CHAPTER 6: NAVIGATING CHALLENGES (CONT.) — **PG#**

I'm lactose intolerant. What do I do?	50-51
If the scale isn't moving, how do I know it's working?	51
I'm not getting into ketosis; what should I do?	51-52
What do I do if I slip up or fall off the wagon?	52
I'm constipated; is this normal?	52-53
How many meals should I eat per day?	53
Can I snack?	53-54
What do I do if my cholesterol gets high?	54

CHAPTER 7: EMBRACING THE KETOGENIC LIFESTYLE — **PG#**

What are "net carbs"?	55
What exactly are MCTs?	55-56
What are exogenous ketones?	56
Will I be able to take breaks?	56-57
I've heard about fasting; should I be doing that too?	57
Are there other keto variations that I can use?	57-58
What can I eat when out with friends or family?	58
Can I drink alcohol while living this way?	58
Does the quality or type of meat & eggs I buy matter?	59-60
Do I need to buy all organic vegetables and fruits?	60-61
Will I have to work out to make this work for me?	61-62
Can I build muscle on the ketogenic diet?	62

OTHER KETOGENIC VARIATIONS

NOTE: Only implement these variations after you have crushed your sugar obsession and become fully keto-adapted.

MACRONUTRIENT-BASED VARIATIONS:

1. Fats = 70% | Protein = 20% | Carbs 10%*
2. Fats = 65% | Protein = 30% | Carbs 5%*
3. Fats = 65% | Protein = 25% | Carbs 10%*
4. Fats = 60% | Protein = 30% | Carbs 10%*

In the initial phase, carbs should be between 20 and 50 grams. Later, adjustments can be made to find your individual carb tolerance.

CARB CYCLING:

Carb cycling is when you introduce more unprocessed or minimally processed carbs into your diet for a set period and then return to your normal ketogenic ratios.

- Higher carbs around daily workout times. (Additional 25 to 50 grams per day, depending on activity level)
- One higher-carb meal per week or once every two weeks.
- Keto for 28 days, then go low-carb for 2 days.
- Keto for 21 days, then go low-carb for the rest of the month.

EXAMPLE DAILY MEAL PLANS

EXAMPLE 1: 2 MEALS PER DAY = 1862 CALORIES

MORNING COFFEE - 149 CALORIES:
- 8 to 12 oz organic black coffee
- ½ to 1 tbsp of keto-approved sweetener of your choice
- ½ tbsp MCT oil
- ½ tbsp heavy cream
- ½ scoop collagen peptides

Fat = 12.1g | Protein = 9.4g | Carbs = 0g
Fat = 74% | Protein = 26% | Carbs = 0%

MEAL 1 - 959 CALORIES:
- 1 Angus 75/25 ground chuck beef pattie
- 1 slice white cheddar cheese
- 3 slices uncured bacon
- 1 oz pork rinds
- 2 oz tomatoes, 1 oz for each slice, and use as your bun
- 1½ tbsp avocado oil mayo
- ½ tbsp mustard
- ½ tbsp no-sugar added ketchup

Fat = 83.4g | Protein = 52.3g | Carbs = 4.9g
Fat = 77% | Protein = 21% | Carbs = 2%

MEAL 2 - 754 CALORIES:
- 4.5 oz ahi tuna grilled in an air-fryer
- 1 tbsp grass-fed butter mixed with 1 tbsp ghee to cook in or use half to cook with, then pour over remaining after cooked
- 6 spears asparagus
- 1 tbsp olive oil for the asparagus
- 2 tsp grated parmesan mixed with Italian or basil seasoning as a topper for asparagus
- 1 cup lettuce, romaine, red cabbage mix
- 1 tbsp hemp hearts
- 2 tbsp grated parmesan cheese
- ½ cup cherry tomatoes
- ½ mini cucumber diced
- 1 tbsp olive oil and vinegar dressing

Fat = 58.4g | Protein = 50.2g | Carbs = 8.9g
Fat = 69% | Protein = 26% | Carbs = 5%

EXAMPLE 2: 3 MEALS PER DAY = 1953 CALORIES

MORNING COFFEE - 91 Calories:
- 8 to 12 oz organic black coffee
- ½ to 1 tbsp of keto-approved sweetener of your choice
- ½ tbsp MCT oil
- ½ tbsp heavy cream

Fat = 9.6g | Protein = 0.4g | Carbs = 0g
Fat = 98% | Protein = 2% | Carbs = 0%

MEAL 1 - 753 CALORIES:
- 3 scrambled eggs with 1 tbsp of heavy cream mixed in
- 1 tbsp of grass-fed butter (melt in the pan before scrambling)
- 2 oz fajita steak
- 1.5 oz avocado
- 1 tbsp sour cream
- ½ tbsp of salsa

- Keto milk (2 ozs of heavy cream & 6 ozs of unsweetened almond or coconut milk)

Fat = 65.4g | Protein = 33.4g | Carbs = 6.5g
Fat = 79% | Protein = 18% | Carbs = 3%

MEAL 2 - 557 CALORIES:
- 1 cup lettuce
- 2 oz grilled chicken
- 1 large boiled egg
- 1 oz shredded cheese
- 1 tbsp hemp hearts
- 5 whisps
- 1 tbsp ranch dressing
- 2 tbsp olive oil and vinegar dressing

Fat = 46.1g | Protein = 31.1g | Carbs = 5.2g
Fat = 74% | Protein = 22% | Carbs = 4%

MEAL 3 - 552 CALORIES:
- 6.5 oz grilled or sauteed shrimp
- 1 tbsp grass-fed butter mixed with 1 tbsp of ghee to cook in or use half to cook with, then pour over remaining after cooked
- ½ cup of zucchini and ¼ cup of mushrooms sauteed
- 1 tbsp of olive oil mixed with ½ tbsp of grass-fed butter to sautee or use half to cook with, then pour over remaining after the veggies are cooked
- ¼ cup blueberries

Fat = 45.7g | Protein = 31.4g | Carbs = 3.4g
Fat = 73% | Protein = 24% | Carbs = 3%

EXAMPLE 3: 4 MEALS PER DAY = 1835 CALORIES

MEAL 1 - 479 CALORIES:
- 8 to 12 oz organic black coffee
- 1 tbsp keto-approved sweetener of your choice
- 2oz heavy cream
- 1 tbsp MCT oil
- 1 scoop vanilla protein powder (IsoPure Zero Carb used here)

Fat = 41.1g | Protein = 25.4g | Carbs = 0g
Fat = 78% | Protein = 22% | Carbs = 0%

MEAL 2 - 570 CALORIES:
- 1 My Fat Yogurt (homemade, recipe in next section)
- ½ oz pecans
- ¼ tsp cinnamon
- 1 large boiled egg
- 1 beef stick (Chomp beef stick used here)

Fat = 46.1g | Protein = 31.1g | Carbs = 5g
Fat = 74% | Protein = 22% | Carbs = 4%

MEAL 3 - 539 CALORIES:
- 5 oz New York strip steak grilled or cooked in an air-fryer
- ½ cup brussels sprouts
- 2 tbsp butter, split between steak and Brussels

Fat = 43.4g | Protein = 30.3g | Carbs = 5.4g
Fat = 73% | Protein = 23% | Carbs = 4%

MEAL 4 - 248 CALORIES:
- ¼ cup whipped cream (homemade, recipe in next section)
- ½ scoop vanilla protein powder (IsoPure Zero Carb used here)
- ½ cup frozen mixed berries (strawberries & blueberries)

Fat = 20.1g | Protein = 12.7g | Carbs = 4.7g
Fat = 72% | Protein = 20% | Carbs = 8%

QUICK & EASY KETO RECIPES

While this isn't a cookbook, I wanted to provide you with a few of my favorite quick recipes to help you get started.

<u>**My Fat Yogurt**</u>
- ¼ cup cottage cheese
- 3 oz low-sugar flavored or plain Greek yogurt
- 2 tbsp MCT oil
- ½ scoop collagen peptides
- 3 drops of liquid organic stevia or ½ packet of powdered

Directions: Combine all the ingredients in a bowl or storage container, stirring well with a spoon until everything is mixed. Cover with a lid and refrigerate. This makes one serving.

Whole Container = 350 Calories
Fat = 30.3g | Protein = 15.3g | Carbs = 3g
Fat = 79% | Protein = 18% | Carbs = 3%

*Add one or several of the following to make it even better:
1 cap full of your favorite sugar-free syrup
½ to 1 oz pecans, walnuts, or macadamia nuts
½ to 1 oz flaked coconut
*Adding any of the above items will change the calories and the macronutrient ratios.

No-Oatsmeal
- 1 cup organic hemp hearts
- ¼ cup organic ground flaxseed
- ¼ cup organic chia seeds
- 1 to 2 tbsp of keto-approved sweetener of your choice
- ½ scoop of protein powder (IsoPure Zero Vanilla used here)
- 8 oz unsweetened coconut milk
- 2 tbsp heavy cream

Directions: You will combine the solids first, then add the powders. You'll want to stir them all together to mix them well. Lastly, put the liquids in and stir well with a fork again until everything is mixed. Put the lid on and place it in the fridge overnight. This will make 2 cups in total, but it can be served in several servings. You can eat a tbsp of or up to half a cup at a time. It can be eaten cold or heated in the microwave for a warm treat.

Whole Container = 1598 Calories:
Fat = 125.4g | Protein = 83.2g | Carbs = 36.2g
Fat = 70% | Protein = 21% | Carbs = 9%

¼ of Container (½ Cup) = 400 Calories:
Fat = 31.3g | Protein = 20.8g | Carbs = 9.1g
Fat = 70% | Protein = 21% | Carbs = 9%

Add one or several of the following to make it even better:
1 cap full of your favorite sugar-free syrup
1 to 2 oz ground nuts; pecans, walnuts, or macadamia
1 to 2 oz flaked coconut
¼ to ½ cup mixed berries
¼ to ½ cup keto-approved fruit
Adding any of the above items will change the calories and the macronutrient ratios.

Homemade Whipped Cream
- ½ cup heavy cream
- 1 to 2 tbsp of keto-approved sweetener of your choice

Directions: You will combine all ingredients in a deep-set glass or metal bowl. You will use a hand mixer on the highest speed for 2 to 4 minutes until it is whipped to your liking.

Whole Container = 360 Calories
Fat = 125.4g | Protein = 83.2g | Carbs = 36.2g
Fat = 70% | Protein = 21% | Carbs = 9%

Add one of several of the following to make it even better:
1 cap full of your favorite sugar-free syrup
1 to 2 oz flaked coconut
¼ to ½ cup mixed berries
¼ to ½ cup keto-approved fruit
Adding any of the above items will change the calories and the macronutrient ratios.

Homemade Cheese Sauce
- 2 tbsp grass-fed salted butter
- 1 oz cream cheese
- ¼ cup heavy cream
- 1 oz unsweetened almond milk
- 4 oz shredded sharp cheddar cheese

Directions: Mix the butter, milk, and heavy cream in a small saucepan on medium heat. Microwave the cream cheese for 8 to 10 seconds, then add it to the liquid once it is at a slight boil. Reduce heat, and add the shredded cheese about 1 oz at a time until done.

Whole Container = 916 Calories
Fat = 87.5g | Protein = 25.3g | Carbs = 2g
Fat = 88% | Protein = 11% | Carbs = 1%

Quick Keto Bread Round
- 3 tbsp blanched almond flour
- 1 tsp Psyllium husk powder
- ½ tsp gluten-free baking powder
- 1 large egg
- 1 tbsp grass-fed salted butter
- ½ tbsp ghee
- ¼ tbsp olive oil
- Pinch of salt of your choice

Directions: You will spray olive oil on the inside of a round glass container. I have found that the 2-cup size works best. Next, you will add the dry ingredients together and mix thoroughly with a fork. Mix butter and ghee in another glass container. Put in the microwave until butter is melted (approx 20 secs). After this has cooled, crack the egg into the container with the butter and ghee, beat until mixed, then add to the dry ingredients bowl. Mix thoroughly until all dry and wet have bonded together. Put into microwave for 90 seconds, release with a fork, then flip over and microwave for another 30 seconds. Let cool for 1 minute, then slice in half.

1 Keto Bread Round = 405 Calories
Fat = 37.3g | Protein = 10.8g | Carbs = 8.8g
Fat = 81% | Protein = 10% | Carbs = 8%

Ground Beef Casserole
- 1 lb 80/20 grass-fed ground beef, season to your liking
- 1 cup organic mixed vegetables
- 3 tsp of minced garlic in olive oil

Directions: Heat garlic and oil until sizzling. Add meat and cook until browned. Next, add the frozen veggies and continue cooking until thoroughly cooked.

Whole Container = 1273 Calories
Fat = 97.8g | Protein = 83.7g | Carbs = 11.8g
Fat = 70% | Protein = 27% | Carbs = 4%

Bison & Chicken Sausage Meatballs

- 1 lb ground bison, season to your liking
- 4 links ground tomato and basil chicken sausage
- 4 oz shredded cheese (parmesan or blend works best)
- 4 oz heavy cream
- 2 large eggs
- 1 tbsp of olive oil

1 Meatball = 142 Calories (Type of cheese used can change this)
Fat = 9.7g | Protein = 12.1g | Carbs = 1.3g
Fat = 62% | Protein = 34% | Carbs = 4%

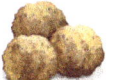

Ground Beef & Italian Sausage Meatballs

- 1 lb 80/20 ground beef, season to your liking
- 1 lb Italian ground beef sausage
- 4 oz shredded cheese (parmesan or blend works best)
- 4 oz heavy cream
- 2 large eggs
- 1 tbsp of olive oil

1 Meatball = 182 Calories (Type of cheese used can change this)
Fat = 15.5g | Protein = 9.7g | Carbs = 0.6g
Fat = 77% | Protein = 22% | Carbs = 1%

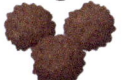

Directions: Start by preheating the oven to 375 degrees. You will want to grind the sausage first if it is not purchased ground. Mix all meat in a large bowl or food processor. Mix the eggs, heavy cream, and cheese in a separate bowl with a large fork; once mixed well, pour the mix over the meat and mix evenly. Once mixed thoroughly, you will want to oil your hands and use a quarter cup measuring cup to measure each meatball; it should be approximately 2 oz each. You will want to roll each meatball and place it on a nonstick cooking mat or parchment paper-lined cookie sheet. The recipe will make between 15 and 18 meatballs. Put in the oven for about 30 minutes; every oven varies, so please watch them.

Breakfast Egg Bites

- 12 large eggs
- 6 tbsp heavy cream
- 3 tbsp grass-fed salted butter
- 1.5 oz Mexican cheese blend
- 6 slices nitrate-free uncured bacon
- 2 oz sweet peppers and/or onions
- Seasonings of your choice

1 Egg Bit = 311 Calories
Fat = 25.3g | Protein = 17.2g | Carbs = 1.5g
Fat = 75% | Protein = 23% | Carbs = 2%

Directions: Start by preheating your oven to 350 degrees. Grease your 6-cup cupcake pan with oil. Pre-cook the bacon in the oven or on the stovetop, whichever you prefer. Once it's cooled, chop it up. I find that oven-cooking bacon on a flat sheet with parchment paper is the easiest and least messy method. If you're using peppers and onions, either get them pre-chopped or cut them yourself before mixing. Melt the butter, then set it aside. Crack all the eggs into a large mixing bowl, and add the heavy cream, cooled butter, and cheese. You can mix it by hand with a fork or use a hand mixer on the lowest setting. Once it's mixed, pour it evenly into the pre-oiled six-large cupcake pan. Now, add your bacon and peppers; we do this at the end instead of mixing in because they tend to go to the bottom, and we want to ensure we get the right amounts in each egg bite. You'll add half an ounce of peppers and onions to each cup. Lastly, you'll put it in the oven for approximately 25 minutes. I suggest checking after about 15 minutes, then again every 5 minutes after that until they are cooked to your liking.

Add one or several of the following to make it even better:
3 oz pork or beef ground sausage
3 oz keto-approved vegetables of your choice
Use some toppings to add even more flavor: cream cheese, avocado, salsa, extra cheese
*Adding any of the above items will change the calories and the macronutrient ratios.

OTHER RESOURCES

Book Resources (Also References):
- The Art And Science Of Low Carbohydrate Living - Written by Jeff S Volek, PhD, RD & Stephen D Phinney, MD, PhD
- Grain Brain - Written by Dr David Perlmutter
- The Real Meal Revolution - Written by Professor Tim Noakes, Jonno Proudfoot & Sally-Ann Creed
- Keto Clarity - Written by Jimmy Moore & Eric C Westman, MD
- Women, Food and Hormones - Written by Sara Gottfried, MD
- Lies My Doctor Told Me - Written by Ken D Berry, MD, FAAFP
- The New Atkins For The New You - Written by Eric C Westman, MD, Stephen D Phinney, MD & Jeff S Volek, PhD
- The Big Fat Surprise - Written by Nina Teicholz
- Pure, White and Deadly (3rd Edition) - Written by John Yukin
- Why We Get Fat - Written by Gary Taubes
- The Banting Pocket Guide - Written by Professor Tim Noakes, Bernadine Douglas & Bridgette Allan
- Cholesterol Clarity - Written by Jimmy Moore & Eric C Westman, MD

Website Resources (Also References):
https://www.cdc.gov/
https://www.who.int/
https://www.healthline.com/

Website Resources (Continued):

https://www.clinicaltrials.gov/
https://www.mayoclinic.org/
https://www.hopkinsmedicine.org/the-johns-hopkins-hospital
https://thenoakesfoundation.org/
https://www.virtahealth.com/
https://ericwestmanmd.com/
https://ketonutrition.org/
https://brainenergy.com/
https://drperlmutter.com/
https://baszuckigroup.com/
https://www.metabolicmind.org/
https://neuroketo.org/
https://garytaubes.com/
https://ninateicholz.com/
https://cholesterolcode.com/

Other Resources (Also References):

- The Metabolic Link - podcast & YouTube channel
- LowCarbUSA - website & YouTube channel
- Low Carb Down Under - website & YouTube channel
- The Metabolic Mind - website & YouTube channel
- Diet Doctor - website & app for keto, low carb, and fasting
- My Fitness Pal - website & app for food tracking
- Cronometer - website & app for food tracking
- Lose It - website & app for food tracking
- Zero - app for information about fasting and fasting tracker
- Audacious Nutrition - resource for exogenous ketones
- HVMN - resource for exogenous ketones

Research Review Resources (Also References):

2020 - Ketogenic Metabolic Therapy Research Review
2021 - Ketogenic Metabolic Therapy Research Review
2022 - Ketogenic Metabolic Therapy Research Review

The Metabolic Health Initiative (MHI) published the above research reviews. They can be obtained with a paid membership, which you can access at: https://membership.metabolicinitiative.com/home

REFERENCES

[JumpstartMD]. (2013, May 17). JumpstartMD Full Interview with Drs. Stephen Phinney & Jeff Volek [Video]. YouTube. https://www.youtube.com/watch?v=OFD2q5iqevY

McAuliffe, L. (2023, December 3). The Keto Diet and Human Evolution. Dr. Robert Kiltz. https://www.doctorkiltz.com/

Schaeffer, J. (2019, April 1). Evolutionary Eating — What We Can Learn From Our Primitive Past. Today's Dietitian Vol. 11 No. 4 P. 36 The Magazine For Nutrition Professionals. https://www.todaysdietitian.com/

Diabetes.co.uk (2019, January 15). Diabetes History. Diabetes.co.uk - The Global Diabetes Community. https://www.diabetes.co.uk/

Rollo M.D., J. (1797). An Account Of Two Cases Of The Diabetes Mellitus With Remarks. The Medical Repository - Annals of Medicine, pgs85-105 https://www.ncbi.nlm.nih.gov/pmc/articles/PMC5112440/

Pillay, J. (2017, January 1). Banting Letter on Corpulence by William Banting 1869 - In Today's English. https://thenoakesfoundation.org/banting-letter-on-corpulence-in-todays-english/

Banting, W. (1993). Letter on Corpulence, Addressed to the Public. Obesity Research, 1(2), 153-163. https://doi.org/10.1002/j.1550-8528.1993.tb00605.x

Barry Groves PhD (2002, September 7). WILLIAM BANTING: The Father of the Low-Carbohydrate Diet. Second Opinions. http://www.second-opinions.co.uk/banting.html

Stefansson, V. (2016). Not by Bread Alone - Eating Meat and Fat for Stay Lean and Healthy. Italy: Youcanprint.

Wheless, J. W. (2008). History of the ketogenic diet. Epilepsia, 49, 3-5. https://doi.org/10.1111/j.1528-1167.2008.01821.x

Stylianou, C., & Kelnar, C. (2009). The introduction of successful treatment of diabetes mellitus with insulin. Journal of the Royal Society of Medicine, 102(7), 298-303. https://doi.org/10.1258/jrsm.2009.09k035

Tran, Q., Lee, H., Kim, C., Kong, G., Gong, N., Kwon, S. H., Park, J., Kim, H., & Park, J. (2020). Revisiting the Warburg Effect: Diet-Based Strategies for Cancer Prevention. BioMed Research International, 2020. https://doi.org/10.1155/2020/8105735

Donaldson, M.D., B. F. (1962). Strong Medicine (1st ed.). Doubleday & Company, Inc.

Leith, W. (1961). Experiences with the Pennington Diet in the Management of Obesity. Canadian Medical Association Journal, 84(25), 1411-1414. https://www.ncbi.nlm.nih.gov/pmc/articles/PMC1848046/

Heffernan, C. (2023, August 16). The History of Vince Gironda, Low Carb Pioneer and Bodybuilding Great. Barbend.com. https://barbend.com/vince-gironda-history/

Atkins (n.d.). Atkins' History. Atkins.com. https://www.atkins.com/our-story/atkins-diet-history#primary

Leslie, I. (2016, April 7). The sugar conspiracy. The Guardian. https://www.theguardian.com/society/2016/apr/07/the-sugar-conspiracy-robert-lustig-john-yudkin

Charlie Foundation (n.d.). Our Story. Charlie Foundation For Ketogenic Therapies. https://charliefoundation.org/about-the-charlie-foundation-for-ketogenic-therapies/

Taubes, G. (2002, July 7). What if It's All Been a Big Fat Lie? The New York Times, Section 6, Pg 22. https://www.nytimes.com/2002/07/07/magazine/what-if-its-all-been-a-big-fat-lie.html

National Library of Medicine (n.d.). Clinical Trials. ClinicalTrials.gov. https://clinicaltrials.gov/

Stone, W. (2024, January 27). Patients say keto helps with their mental illness. Science is racing to understand why. Npr.org. https://www.npr.org/sections/health-shots/2024/01/27/1227062470/ketokogenic-diet-mental-illness-bipolar-depression

International Neurological Ketogenic Society (n.d.). Keto Research Papers 2023. Neuroketo.org. https://neuroketo.org/links-and-resources/keto-research-papers-2022/

FDA (2022, August 8). Development & Approval Process | Drugs. U.S. Food & Drug Administration. https://www.fda.gov/drugs/development-approval-process-drugs

Virta Health (n.d.). Stephen Phinney, MD, PhD Founder, former Chief Medical Officer, current Virta Advisor. Virtahealth.com. https://www.virtahealth.com/people/stephen-phinney

The Noakes Foundation (n.d.). Prof Tim Noakes. Thenoakesfoundation.org. https://thenoakesfoundation.org/prof-tim-noakes/

The Ohio State University (n.d.). Jeff Volek Biography. Ehe.osu.edu. https://ehe.osu.edu/directory?id=volek.1

Duke Health (n.d.). Eric C. Westman, MD, MHS. Dukehealth.org. https://www.dukehealth.org/find-doctors-physicians/eric-c-westman-md-mhs

USF Health (n.d.). Molecular Pharmacology and Physiology Faculty Dominic D'Agostino, Ph.D. Health.usf.edu. https://health.usf.edu/medicine/mpp/faculty/ddagosti

Chris Palmer, M.D. (n.d.). Chris Palmer MD - About Dr Palmer. Chrispalmermd.com. https://www.chrispalmermd.com/chris-palmer/

WHO (2024, March 1). Obesity and overweight. World Health Organization. https://www.who.int/news-room/fact-sheets/detail/obesity-and-overweight

Ahmad FB, Cisewski JA, Xu J, Anderson RN. Provisional Mortality Data — (2022). MMWR Morb Mortal Wkly Rep 2023;72:488–492. DOI: http://dx.doi.org/10.15585/mmwr.mm7218a3

CDC (2024, February 5). Obesity, Race/Ethnicity, and COVID-19. Centers For Disease Control And Prevention. https://www.cdc.gov/obesity/data/obesity-and-covid-19.html

Perlmutter MD, D. (2019). Grain Brain (3rd ed.). Yellow Kite. https://drperlmutter.com/books/grain-brain-by-david-perlmutter/

CDC (2022, October 25). By the Numbers: Diabetes in America Source: National Diabetes Statistics Report, 2023. Centers for Disease Control and Prevention. https://www.cdc.gov/diabetes/health-equity/diabetes-by-the-numbers.html

Virta Health (n.d.). About Virta. Virta. https://www.virtahealth.com/about

Ayonrinde, O. T. (2021). Historical narrative from fatty liver in the nineteenth century to contemporary NAFLD – Reconciling the present with the past. JHEP Reports, 3(3), 100261. https://doi.org/10.1016/j.jhepr.2021.100261

American Liver Foundation (2024, March 7). Nonalcoholic Fatty Liver Disease (NAFLD). Liverfoundation.org. https://liverfoundation.org/liver-diseases/fatty-liver-disease/nonalcoholic-fatty-liver-disease-nafld/

National Institutes of Health (2021, December). Symptoms & Causes of NAFLD & NASH in Children. National Institute of Diabetes and Digestive and Kidney Diseases (NIDDK). https://www.niddk.nih.gov/health-information/liver-disease/nafld-nash-children/symptoms-causes

Witters, D. (2023, May 17). U.S. Depression Rates Reach New Highs. Gallup https://news.gallup.com/poll/505745/depression-rates-reach-new-highs.aspx

Palmer, MD, C. M. (2022). Brain Energy (1st ed.). BenBella Books, Inc. https://brainenergy.com/

Palmer, C. M. (2017). Ketogenic diet in the treatment of schizoaffective disorder: Two case studies. Schizophrenia Research, 189, 208-209. https://doi.org/10.1016/j.schres.2017.01.053

Ede MD, G. (2022, July 19). New Study: Serious Mental Illness Improves on Ketogenic Diet. Psychology Today. https://www.psychologytoday.com/us/blog/diagnosis-diet/202207/new-study-serious-mental-illness-improves-ketogenic-diet

[Low Carb Down Under]. (2022, January 21). Dr. Stephen Phinney - 'The Realities of Sustained Nutritional Ketosis' [Video]. YouTube. https://www.youtube.com/watch?v=Hs0zzox-TF0

Horton, MS, RD, B., & Pallarito, K. (2024, January 3). The 25 Best Low-Carb, Keto-Friendly Beers. Health.com. https://www.health.com/weight-loss/best-low-carb-beer-keto

Gaedke, M. (n.d.). 15 Best Wines for Keto. Ketoconnect.net. https://www.ketoconnect.net/best-wines-for-keto/

Quezada, N. (2023). Terrible vs Great [Photograph]. Understanding Food Labels Presentation.

National Institute on Aging (2022, February 24). How To Read Food and Beverage Labels. Nia.nih.gov. https://www.nia.nih.gov/health/healthy-eating-nutrition-and-diet/how-read-food-and-beverage-labels

O'Donnell, M., Mente, A., Rangarajan, S., McQueen, M. J., Wang, X., Liu, L., ... & Yusuf, S. (2014). [Photograph]. Urinary sodium and potassium excretion, mortality, and cardiovascular events. New England Journal of Medicine, 371(7), 612-623.

Ajmera, MS, RD, R., & Spritzler, F. (2023, December 6). 12 Evidence-Based Health Benefits of Magnesium. Healthline.com. https://www.healthline.com/nutrition/magnesium-benefits

Farm Aid (n.d.). Food Labels Explained. Farmaid.org. https://www.farmaid.org/food-labels-explained/

Environmental Work Group (2024, March 20). EWGs Dirty Dozen and Clean Fifteen Lists. Ewg.org. https://www.ewg.org/

ABOUT THE AUTHOR

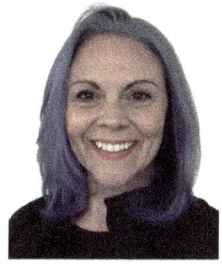

Nicole is a dedicated advocate for nutrition, health, and wellness, with a passion for helping others transform their lives. After years of struggling with focus, memory, and weight issues in her thirties—and finding little relief through conventional medicine—Nicole took control of her own health. This personal journey led her to explore holistic healing through nutrition, mindfulness, gratitude, and movement.

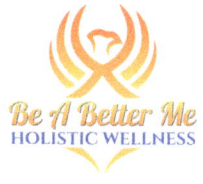

Now a highly sought-after nutrition coach and elite-certified personal trainer, Nicole holds multiple certifications in nutrition, health sciences, and behavioral change. She specializes in low-carb and ketogenic lifestyles, guiding her clients toward healthier, happier, and more fulfilling lives. Through her coaching and teaching, Nicole empowers others to achieve lasting wellness and joy.

- @colorfulketo
- @beabetterme.today
- @beabetterme.today
- www.beabettermetoday.com
- nicole@beabettermetoday.com

www.ingramcontent.com/pod-product-compliance
Lightning Source LLC
Chambersburg PA
CBHW070527030426
42337CB00016B/2139